HAND-BOOK OF HYGIENIC PRACTICE

(1864)

INTENDED AS A PRACTICAL GUIDE FOR THE SICK ROOM

> "No person can prescribe for the sick very satisfactorily, nor with the success which is due to the true Art of healing, without a general knowledge of the fundamental principles or ground work of the system which he presumes to practice. The curative agents of the Hygienic Medical System are normal materials and influences, in contradiction to those of all Drug Medical Systems which are abnormal, or in other words, toxicological, morbific poisons."

R.T. Trall

ISBN 1-56459-807-1

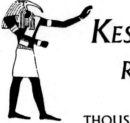
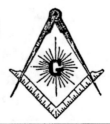

Warning—Disclaimer

PREFACE.

Twenty years' experience in the practice of the Hygienic System, and a dozen years' observation in teaching the system to classes of medical students, have enabled us to see very clearly, what is needed in the way of Hygienic medical literature, in order to establish the system on an enduring basis, and ensure to the human race the inestimable blessings which the recognition of its principles and perfection of its practice are calculated to confer. The great masses of the people have neither time, opportunity, nor inclination to investigate intricate medical problems, nor to search out first principles. While they are in health they do not see nor feel the necessity nor importance of so doing, and when they are sick they are to a great extent, unfitted for the task. Hence the need of plain rules for self-treatment, and specific directions for administering the remedial appliances of our system of the Healing Art at the bedside of the patient. For such this work is intended. For another class, who are destined to be the leaders and pioneers in the GREAT HEALTH REFORM MOVEMENT, and for all who desire to be self-educated in the whole Philosophy of Medical Science, and especially for those who propose to be Teachers and Practitioners of Hygeio-Therapy, I am preparing, and have nearly completed, a large and elaborate work, entitled, "Principles of Hygienic Medication," which will be a complete exposition of all medical doctrines and systems, and a full explanation and illustration of all the Primary Problems of Medical Science and the Healing Art.

If any apology is needed for the long delay in putting this work to press, since it was announced as forthcoming, I can only plead multitudinous and engrossing professional duties. The medical direction of two Hygienic Institutions constantly thronged with invalids; a large office practice; an extensive correspondence; the sole care and management of the New York Hygeio-Therapeutic College, and of the HERALD OF HEALTH, with occasional popular lectures, have so occupied my time, as to render book-making nearly a business of odd moments and midnight toil.

                                                    R. T. T.

NEW YORK, 1864.

INTRODUCTION.

No PERSON can prescribe for the sick very satisfactorily, nor with the success which is due to the true Art of Healing, without a general knowledge of the fundamental principles or ground-work of the system which he presumes to practice. The curative agents of the Hygienic Medical System (improperly called Hydropathy, or Water-Cure,) are *normal* materials and influences, in contradiction to those of all Drug Medical Systems which are *abnormal*, or in other words, toxicological, morbific—poisons.

The following explanations are copied substantially from my prescription circulars, and from a small work I have published entitled, " Water-Cure for the Million."

PRINCIPLES OF HYGIENIC MEDICATION.

ALL healing power is inherent in the living system.

There is no curative " virtue" in medicines, nor in anything outside the vital organism.

Nature has not provided remedies for diseases.

There is no " law of cure" in the universe ; and the only condition of cure is, obedience to physiological law.

Remedial agents do not act on the living system, as taught in medical books and schools, but are *acted on* by the vital powers.

Disease is not, as is commonly supposed, an enemy at war with the vital powers, but a remedial effort—a process of purification and reparation. It is not a *thing* to be destroyed, subdued, or suppressed, but an *action* to be *regulated* and *directed*.

Truly remedial agents are materials and influences which have *normal* relations to the vital organs, and not drugs, or poisons, whose relations are *abnormal* and *anti-vital*.

Nature's *materia medica* consists of *Air, Light, Temperature, Electricity, Magnetism, Exercise, Rest, Food, Drink, Bathing, Sleep, Clothing, Passional Influences,* and *Mechanical or Surgical Appliances*.

The True Healing Art consists in supplying the living system with whatever of the above it can *use* under the circumstances, and not in the administration of poisons which it must *resist* and *expel*.

Drug remedies are themselves *causes* of disease. If they cure one disease, it is only by producing a drug disease. Every dose diminishes the vitality of the patient.

Drugopathy endeavors to restore health by administering the poisons which produce disease.

Hygeio-Therapy (erroneously called "Hydropathy," or "Water-Cure,") on the contrary, restores the sick to health by the means which preserve health in well persons.

Diseases are caused by obstructions, the obstructing materials being poisons or impurities of some kind.

The Hygienic system removes these obstructions, and leaves the body sound.

Drug medicines add to the causes of obstructions, and change acute into chronic diseases.

To attempt to cure diseases by adding to the causes of disease, is irrational and absurd.

Hygienic medication (Hygeio-Therapy) is not a one-ideaism which professes to cure all diseases with "water alone." Nor is it a "*Cold* Water-Cure," as is erroneously believed by many. It adopts all the remedial appliances in existence, with the single exception of *poisons*.

BATHING PROCESSES.

WET SHEET PACKING.—On a bed or mattress two or three comfortables or bed-quilts are spread; over them a pair of flannel blankets; and lastly, a wet sheet (rather coarse linen is best) wrung out lightly. The patient, undressed, lies down flat on the back, and is quickly enveloped in the sheet, blanket, and other bedding. The head must be well raised with pillows, and care must be taken to have the feet well wrapped. If the feet do not warm with the rest of the body, a jug of hot water should be applied; and if there is tendency to headache, several folds of cold wet cloth should be laid over the forehead. The usual time for remaining in the pack is from forty to sixty minutes. It may be followed by the plunge, half-bath, rubbing wet sheet, or towel wash, according to circumstances. The pack is not intended as a sweating process, as many suppose, though a moderate perspiration is not objectionable. A comfortable temperature of the surface is the desideratum, independent of more or less sweating, or none at all. When the patient warms up rapidly, thirty minutes or less will be long enough to remain enveloped; but when he becomes warm slowly and with difficulty, an hour, or more, is not too long. In some cases it is necessary to put hot bottles to the sides as well as to the feet. When the object is to cool a fever, the sheet should be allowed to retain more water, or if the skin is very hot, double sheets may be used. In chronic diseases, when the main object is to induce "reaction," or rather circulation, toward the surface, the sheet should be wrung more thoroughly, and the patient enveloped with a greater quantity of blankets, comfortables, or other bedding.

HALF-PACK.—This is the same as the preceding, with the exception that the neck and extremities are not covered by the wet sheet, which is applied merely to the trunk of the body, from the armpits to the hips. It is adapted to those whose circulation is too feeble for a full pack ; it is also often appropriately employed as a preparation for the full pack.

HALF-BATH.—An oval or oblong tub is most convenient, though any vessel allowing a patient to sit down with the legs extended will answer. The water should cover the lower extremities and about half of the abdomen. While in the bath, the patient, if able, should rub the lower extremities, while the attendant rubs the chest, back, and abdomen.

HIP OR SITZ-BATH.—Any small-sized wash-tub will do for this, although tubs constructed with a straight back, and raised four or five inches from the floor, are much the most agreeable. The water should just cover the hips and lower part of the abdomen. A blanket should be thrown over the patient, who will find it also useful to rub or knead the abdomen with the hand or fingers during the bath.

FOOT-BATH.—Any small vessel, as a pail, will answer. Usually the water should be about ankle-deep ; but very delicate invalids, or extremely susceptible persons, should not have the water more than half an inch to one inch in depth. During the bath, the feet should be kept in gentle motion. Walking foot-baths are excellent in warm weather, where a cool stream can be found.

HOT AND COLD FOOT-BATH.—Place the feet in water as warm as can be borne for five or ten minutes ; then dip them for a moment in cold water, and wipe dry.

RUBBING WET-SHEET.—If the sheet is used *drippingly* wet, the patient stands in the tub ; if wrung so as not to drip, the patient may stand on a carpet or on the floor. The sheet is thrown around the body, which it completely envelops below the neck ; the attendant rubs the body over the sheet (not with it), the patient exercising himself at the same time by rubbing in front.

PAIL-DOUCHE.—This means simply pouring water over the chest and shoulders from a pail.

STREAM-DOUCHE.—A stream of water may be applied to the part or parts affected, by pouring from a pitcher or other convenient vessel, held as high as possible; or a barrel or keg may be elevated for the purpose, having a tube of any desired size. The power will be proportional to the amount of water in the reservoir.

a small cask/ barrel

TOWEL OR SPONGE BATH.—Rubbing the whole surface with a coarse wet towel or sponge, followed by a dry sheet or towels, constitutes this process.

AFFUSION BATH.—This implies pouring water gently over the surface of the body. The patient may stand in a tub, or lie on the bed, the bedding being protected by a sheet of India-rubber or gutta-percha.

THE PLUNGE-BATH.—This is employed but little, except at the establishments. Those who have conveniences will often find it one of the best processes. Any tub or box holding water enough to allow the whole body to be immersed, with limbs extended, answers the purpose. A very good plunge can be made of a large cask cut in two near the middle. It is a useful precaution to wet the head before taking this bath.

DROP-BATH.—A vessel, filled with *very cold* water, is furnished with a small aperture through which the water falls in drops. It is adapted to torpid muscles, paralytic limbs, tumors, etc. It should be followed by active friction.

opening/hole

having lost motion/power of exertion

THE SWEATING-PACK.—To produce perspiration, the patient is packed in the flannel blanket and other bedding, as mentioned above, omitting the wet sheet. Some will perspire in less than an hour; others require several hours. This is the severest of the Water-Cure processes, and in fact, is very seldom called for. The warm, hot, or vapor-baths are, in most cases, preferable.

HEAD-BATH.—The patient lies extended on a rug or mattress, the head resting in a shallow basin or bowl, holding two or three inches of water, the shoulders being supported by a pillow. It is principally employed in chronic affections of the head, eyes, and ears. Wet cloths applied to the head, the "pouring-bath," and the "wet cap" are good substitutes.

THE POURING HEAD-BATH.—The patient lies face downward, the head supported by an attendant, projecting over the side of the bed, which is protected by a sheet or blanket thrown around the patient's neck; a tub is placed under the head to catch the water, which is poured from a pitcher moderately, but steadily, for several minutes, or until the head is well cooled, the stream being principally applied to the temples and back part of the head. It is useful in severe cases of sick headache; in the early stage of violent choleras; in the early stages of fevers, when attended with great gastric irritation or biliary disturbance. In hysteria, apoplexy, delirum-tremens, nose-bleeding, inflammation of the brain, ophthalmia, otitis, etc., it has been employed with advantage.

FOUNTAIN, OR SPRAY-BATH.—This consists of a number of small streams of water directed to a particular part of the body. It may be regarded as a gentle douche or local shower. It is intended to excite action and promote absorption in the part or organ to which it is applied.

THE SHOWER-BATH.—This needs no description. It is not frequently used in Water-Cure, but is often very convenient. Those liable to a "rush of blood to the head," should not allow much of the shock of the stream upon the head. Feeble persons should never use this bath until prepared by other treatment. Placing the feet for a few minutes in warm water, before taking the shower, is a good preparatory measure for feeble persons. Standing in warm water, ankle deep, will materially lessen its shock on the brain and nervous system.

NASAL, MOUTH, AND EYE BATHS.—Drawing water gently up the nostrils and ejecting it by the mouth, holding water in the mouth, and holding the eyes open in water of a temperature suited to the case, are the processes indicated by these terms. They are useful in relaxed and inflammatory affections of the mucous membranes and other structures of the parts.

ARM AND LEG BATHS.—The limbs may be held in any convenient vessel containing the requisite depth of water. These baths are useful in cases of fever sores, chronic ulcers, inflammatory affections of the joints, etc.

VAPOR-BATH.—Hot stones or bricks may be employed to generate vapor or steam. The patient may sit naked on an open-work chair, with blankets pinned around the neck; a small tub or a common tin-pan, holding a quart of water, is placed under the chair, and red-hot bricks or stones occasionally put in the vessel, so as to keep the vapor constantly rising from the surface of the water. Another very simple plan is this: Procure a one-gallon tin boiler, with a half-inch tin-pipe, having two or three joints and a single elbow. The boiler may be heated on any ordinary stove, grate, or furnace, and the pipe so attached to it as to convey the steam under the chair in which the patient sits, covered from the neck downward with blankets. It may be employed from ten to thirty minutes, according to the amount of vapor generated.

AIR-BATH.—The whole body is suddenly exposed to cool or cold air, or even to a strong current, and an excellent and invigorating process it is in many cases. There is no danger from it, provided the surface has a comfortable glow or temperature at the time, and the circulation is maintained by active exercise. Friction with the hand, a sheet, towel, or flesh-brush, is beneficial at the same time.

BANDAGES AND COMPRESSES.—These are wet cloths, applied to any weak, sore, hot, painful, or diseased part, and renewed as often as they become dry or very warm. The best surgeons have, in all ages, employed "water dressings" alone in local wounds, injuries, and inflammations. They may be *warming* or *cooling* to the part, as they are covered, or not, with dry cloths.

THE WET-GIRDLE.—Three or four yards of crash toweling make a good one. One half of it is wet and applied around the abdomen, followed by the dry half to cover it. It should be wetted so often as it becomes dry. It is extensively employed in bilious and dyspeptic affections, female weaknesses, etc. When required to be worn for a long time, it should, after the first few weeks, be omitted occasionally, or worn only a part of each day, so that the skin over which it is applied will not become too tender. It should not be worn when it occasions permanent chilliness.

THE CHEST-WRAPPER.—This is made of coarse linen, to fit the trunk like an under-shirt, from the neck to the lower ribs; it is applied as wet as possible without dripping, and covered by a similar dry wrapper, made of Canton or light woolen flannel. It requires renewing two or three times a day. It is useful in most cases of pneumonia, asthma, consumption, bronchitis, etc. The same precautions apply to its prolonged employment as mentioned under the head of the wet girdle.

FOMENTATIONS.—These are employed for relaxing muscles, relieving spasms, griping, nervous headache, etc. Any cloths wet in hot water and applied as warm as can be borne, generally answer the purpose; but flannel cloths dipped in hot water, and wrung nearly dry in another cloth or handkerchief, so as to steam the part moderately, are the most efficient sedatives. They are usually employed from five to fifteen minutes. They are useful in cases of severe constipation, colic, dysmenorrhea, hysteria, etc.

REFRIGERATION.—One part of common salt to two parts of snow or pounded ice makes a good freezing mixture. It is inclosed in a very thin cloth, and applied for a few minutes, until the requisite degree of congelation has taken place. It is useful in felons, styes, malignant tumors and ulcers, fever sores, cancers, and in some forms of neuralgia and rheumatism.

WET-DRESS BATH.—This is a method of self-packing, enabling the patient to dispense with the services of an attendant. A linen sheet is fashioned into the form of a night-dress, with large sleeves, and after the bed is prepared, the dress can be wet and put on; the patient can then get into bed and wrap himself sufficiently to secure a comfortable reaction.

ELECTRO-CHEMICAL BATH.—A copper-lined bath-tub is necessary for this process. The patient is immersed in warm water up to the neck; one hand is brought in contact with the positive pole of a strong galvanic battery, the negative pole being in contact with the metallic lining of the tub. The water is usually acidulated, though in some cases alkalies are employed. From half a pint to a pint of nitric acid is put into the water for each bath. It should not be mixed with the water until the galvanic circuit is completed, either by having the patient in connection with the poles of the battery, or these in contact with the copper-lining of the bath-tub. The patient may remain in the bath from ten minutes to half an hour. This bath is very useful in a torpid condition of the skin with low circulation; in glandular obstructions; scrofulas, rheumatic and gouty affections; in chronic congestions of the liver, and to aid the elimination of mineral medicines and other poisons.

INJECTIONS.—These are warm or tepid, cool or cold. The former are used to quiet pain and produce free discharges; the latter to check excessive evacuations and strengthen the bowels. For the former purpose as large a quantity should be used as the bowels can conveniently receive; and for the latter purpose only a small quantity—as much as can be conveniently retained. Small enemas of very cold water are highly serviceable in cases of piles, prolapsus, fissures, etc. The self-injecting syringe is the most convenient instrument. With a rectal, vaginal, and intra-uterine tube, it will answer all possible purposes, for old or young, male or female. These articles can all be furnished for $3.

GENERAL BATHING RULES.

NEVER bathe soon after eating. The most powerful baths should be taken when the stomach is most empty. No full bath should be taken less than three hours after a full meal. Great heat or profuse perspiration are no objections to going into cold water, provided the respiration is not disturbed, and the patient is not greatly fatigued or exhausted. The body should always be comfortably warm at the time of taking any cold bath. Exercise, friction, dry wrapping, or fire may be resorted to, according to circumstances. Very feeble persons should commence treatment with warm or tepid water, gradually lowering the temperature. All shocks, such as shower-baths, douches, plunges, etc., should be avoided by very feeble and irritable invalids; by consumptives in the second and later stages; by those who are liable to great local determinations, or congestions, as "rush of blood to the head," bleeding from the stomach or lungs, etc.; in displacements of the bowels or uterus; during the menstrual period of females; during any considerable crisis or critical effort; after the crisis or "turn" of any fever, or other acute disease; during the existence of any powerful emotion or excitement; soon after eating or copious drinking; in all cases attended with profuse discharges, as diarrhea, cholera, diabetes, hemorrhages; during the suppurative stage of extensive abscesses or ulcers. The heat or feverishness which may attend any of the conditions or diseases above-named should always be abated by tepid affusions or spongings. It is dangerous to employ the wet-sheet pack, in prolonged or violent fevers, after the crisis or turn of the fever. Many errors have been committed in ignorance of this rule. Never eat immediately after bathing.

DURATION OF BATHS.

MANY errors are committed by remaining in cold baths for too long a time. I have known cases in which dyspeptics and consumptives, at Water-Cure establishments, were kept in cold sitz-baths for two hours at a time, once or twice a day. This was intended as a derivative measure, but it worked very injuriously for the patients. Derivative baths, like all others, must be determined by the condition of the patient, not by the thermometer nor chronometer. Sitz-baths of a mild temperature should seldom be prolonged beyond twenty minutes; more frequently ten to fifteen minutes are preferable. It is better to repeat all bathing appliances frequently, than to make violent impressions less frequently. Plunges, douches, and showers, if the water is cold or cool, should not ordinarily be continued more than a minute; when the temperature of the water is temperate, or tepid, they may be taken from five to ten minutes. Tepid half-baths should usually be taken from five to ten minutes. Sitz-baths, foot-baths, head-baths, arm and leg baths, etc., may vary from five to thirty minutes. But, as already intimated, regard must always be had to the temperature of the water and the circulation of the patient.

CRISES.

THOSE general disturbances of the system, transfers of morbid action, or aggravations of symptoms, constituting crises, do not occur so frequently nor with so much severity in home-practice as under the more thorough and systematic course at a water-cure. Nevertheless they do occasionally occur; and then all the patient has to do is to moderate the treatment in precise ratio to the violence of the crisis. Keep quiet and cool, taking no more exercise than is agreeable to the feelings, and *let Nature have her course.* After it is over, if the patient is not cured, the treatment may be resumed as before. In some few cases, as in mercurial diseases, gout and rheumatism, the crises may be so violent as to render some part of the body excessively sore and painful; or the whole body feverish, tender, and inflammatory. In these cases one or two full hot-baths, ten to twenty minutes, should be employed.

Crises usually take the form of diarrhea, feverishness, rashes, or boils. Should diarrhea be very severe, it may be soothed by warm hip-baths. Feverishness is relieved by quiet, or a warm bath at bed-time. When rashes or boils become troublesome under the application of wet cloths, these should be omitted until the skin heals. It is a common error with people, and with some Hydropathic physicians, that crises are always essential to a cure. Many cases of the worst kind recover without any critical disturbance whatever. Nor should the practitioner ever aim to produce a crises. If a crisis appear spontaneously in course of the treatment, it indicates a favorable effort of the vital powers, and is always followed by an improvement. But if provoked by excessive bathing, or mal-treatment of any kind, it is more injurious than useful. I have known cases, repeatedly, in which the patients were "under crisis," as it was said, for several months—in one case for two years. Such cases can be cured, by judicious management, in half the time that they are kept "under crisis" by the crisis doctors.

ABRADED AND ULCERATED SURFACES.—The best application to parts where the skin is destroyed, as in ulcers, burns, scalds, rashes, small-pox, erysipelas, and various excoriations, is dry wheaten flour. It should fill the cavities and cover the surface completely so as to exclude the atmospheric air. Applied to burns and scalds instantly, it will stop the pain and prevent vesication—a fact which all families will do well to remember.

TEMPERATURE.

So far as protection from the atmosphere is concerned, the general rule, is to keep the patient as cool as possible consistent with comfort. In cases of burns and scalds, when the surface is destroyed, the pain may be very much mitigated by keeping the temperature of the room as high as the patient can well bear.

In the application of water, for hygienic or for remedial purposes, the invariable rule to guide us is, the temperature and circulation of the patient. The warmer his surface the colder should be the water employed, and *vice versa*. The sensations of the patient should also be consulted. The more feeble and delicate the patient, and the more susceptible his feelings to the shock or impression of cold water, or cold air, the more carefully should we regard his sensations, in the temperature of the baths prescribed. Mischief is frequently done in home-practice, by applying the water too cold. Very cold or very warm baths should be brief, precisely in ratio of their temperature. Tepid baths may be more prolonged. Baths may be regarded as *very cold* when the temperature is forty degrees or below; *cold*, from forty degrees to sixty degrees; *cool*, from sixty to seventy degrees; *temperate*, from seventy to seventy-five degrees; *tepid*, from seventy-five to eighty-five degrees; *warm*, from eighty-five to ninety-eight degrees; *hot*, above ninety-eight. Hot-baths range from ninety-eight to one hundred and fifteen; vapor-baths from ninety-eight to one hundred and twenty-five. For bathing infants and young children the temperature should ordinarily be from seventy-two to eighty-five degrees. The greatest error in home treatment is in giving too many *cold* baths.

WATER-DRINKING.

THIRST is the general rule for water-drinking. Those who use a plain, unstimulating diet have little thirst, and require but little drink. It is injurious to load the stomach with a large quantity of water when nature does not demand it. As with food, all that can not be used is a burden which must be thrown off. The routine practice of drinking so many tumblers per day, as is advised at some water-cures, is very reprehensible. It is well to take a tumbler of water after the morning ablution, and at other times according to thirst. It is unnatural, and hence injurious, to drink at meals. Throughout the whole animal kingdom nature has intended the saliva to be the solvent of the food. If the food is well masticated and insalivated, it will never need any water to "wash it down." In acute diseases there is often extreme thirst; and here water-drinking may be indulged *ad libitum*; but it is better to "take a little and often," than to take large draughts at long intervals. In many cases of low fevers, cholera, etc., warm water will allay thirst better than cold. Enemas of warm water will also check thirst very promptly.

Cool, but not very cold, water is the most natural drink. But it is always important to have the water pure. Hard and impure waters are a prolific source of affections of the liver and kidneys. For invalids it is of especial importance that all the water taken into the stomach be soft and pure. Artificial "mineral waters," and the saline, alkaline, ferruginous, sulphurous compounds of the "medicinal springs," are pernicious beverages for the sick or well. The drugs they contain are no better, and no different in effect, than the same drugs taken from the apothecary shop. Those Water-Cure physicians who *permit* their patients to use them may be justified in thus yielding to popular prejudice; but to *prescribe* them, argues strange ignorance of Hygiene, or perhaps a worse motive.

FOOD.

DIETETIC RULES.—As fruits and farinacea are the natural food of man, preference should always be given to a vegetarian diet, whenever it can be properly prepared. Those who use animal food should never eat of it more than once a day; and they should restrict themselves to the lean flesh of vegetarian animals.

Milk, and its products—butter and cheese—though favorite articles with many invalids, are in no sense physiological or natural food for adults. A large experience in this matter has convinced me that all invalids (except infants and young children) can do much better without them. Eggs, rare-boiled, may be placed in this category.

The best forms of animal food are beef and mutton, broiled or boiled.

Fish, and particularly shell-fish, are among the least nutritious and grossest kinds of animal food.

With regard to condiments of all kinds, salt, sugar, vinegar, pepper, spices, etc., the rule is, the less the better.

Salt is an indigestible mineral substance, and in no sense dietetical. This last is also true of vinegar.

The best seasonings are the saccharine and acid principles of vegetables and fruits, as sugar or syrup, lemon-juice, etc. But even these should be employed in moderation.

Among the fruits particularly recommended to invalids are apples, grapes, pears, peaches, cherries, sweet oranges, tomatoes, prunes, berries in their season, squashes, and pumpkins.

Of the vegetables we may especially commend potatoes, beans, peas, parsneps, asparagus, spinach, green peas, and green corn. Those whose digestive powers are not much impaired, can partake, without detriment, of cabbage, carrots, turnips, and cucumbers.

Invalids, however, in addition to bread and fruit, had better use but one or two vegetables at one meal.

As a general rule, breakfast should consist of bread and

fruit; dinner, of bread and fruit with vegetables; and supper, of bread with a small allowance of fruit.

Those who use animal food should take it at the noon meal. The breakfast should be light, and supper very light. Those who do not use fruit at dinner, may use a greater proportion of vegetables.

Mushes, as wheaten grits, rice, hominy, corn meal, etc., may be used as a part of bread-food, at breakfast or supper. But they should always be eaten with a hard cracker, dry crust, parched corn, or something that will insure due mastication and insalivation.

TIMES OF EATING.—I do not regard it as of very great importance whether we eat once, twice, or thrice a day, provided we are regular in our habits, and have a proper regard for the time between meals, and the quantity and variety of our viands. I have known patients to do very well on a single meal a day. One of my patients—Miss E. M. HURD, of Sparta, N. J.—who afterward became my student, and is now a physician and the wife of Dr. N. W. FALES, of California, lived on one meal a day for more than a year. When she commenced this plan she was an emaciated dyspeptic, but became healthy and fleshy while adhering to it. Another graduate of our school—Dr. E. P. MILLER, now my associate physician in the New York Water-Cure—has eaten but once a day for a long time. He was also badly dyspeptic when he first adopted the plan, but is now as fair a specimen of health and activity as can easily be found.

I have known hundreds to improve rapidly in changing from three meals a day to two. Probably the majority of invalids, and especially those who are decidedly dyspeptic, will find it beneficial to eat but twice. Those who take three meals a day should take breakfast from six to seven, A. M.; dinner, from twelve, M. to one, P. M.; supper, about six, P. M. Those who eat but twice should take breakfast at about eight, A. M., and the other meal at about three, P. M. Those who adopt the one-meal-a-day system, should obviously *feast* about the middle of the day.

PREPARATION OF FOOD.—After all, the most difficult part of the Hygienic system is the management of the dietary. Few persons know anything about hydropathic cooking; and so perverted are the appetences of the masses, that to talk to them of physiological victuals is very much like talking to a brandy-toper of the beauties of "clear cold water," or to a tobacco-smoker of the virtues of a pure atmosphere. Bread, which is, or should be, the staff of life, has, by the perversions of flouring-mills and the bakers, become a prolific source of disease and death. Much as Health Reformers declaim against the abominations of pork, ham, sausages, and lard, as articles of human food, I am of the opinion that fine flour, in its various forms of bread, short-cake, butter-biscuits, doughnuts, puddings, and pastry, is quite as productive of disease as are the grosser elements of the scavenger swine.

Nearly all the bread used in civilized society is made of fine or superfine flour, which is always obstructing and constipating, and which is deficient in some of the most important elements of the grain; and it is still further vitiated by fermentation, or by acids and alkalies which are employed to render the bread light.

Pure and wholesome bread can have but three ingredients —meal, water, and atmospheric air. The water is only useful in converting the meal into dough; and the atmospheric air serves to expand its particles so as to make light and tender bread. If properly managed, bread can be made as light as ordinary loaf-bread with no other rising than atmospheric air. To effect this, three essentials must be regarded. 1. The dough must be mixed to a proper consistence—neither too stiff nor too soft. 2. The dough must be cut or rolled into cakes or pieces so as to expose the greatest possible surface to the heat of the oven. 3. The oven must have a brisk or quick fire. The hotter the oven—provided it does not burn the dough—when the baking process begins, the lighter will be the bread. The reason is this: The heat, when sufficient, instantly forms a nearly impervious crust over the dough, by which the air is retained, and, expanded by the heat of the oven without being able to escape, separates the particles of dough, and thus renders the bread light.

If the meal is mixed with cold water instead of hot, and allowed to stand and swell for several hours before baking, it will be nearly as light as if mixed with hot water and baked at once.

As good bread may be regarded as the great regulator of the patient's dietary, too much pains can not be taken with it. All persons who undertake home-treatment should acquaint themselves with the processes for making it. Bread made in the manner I am about to explain can always be had fresh for each day or each meal, and may be eaten as soon after cooked as sufficiently cooled. It requires but a few minutes of time, and a supply can be made before breakfast for the day. Or a supply can be made for several days. If heated a few minutes, when two or three days old, it has the tenderness and flavor of freshly-made bread. It is still more tender if dipped in cold water and then heated.

BREAD ROLLS.—Mix wheat-meal (Graham flour) with boiling water quickly, by stirring rapidly with a stick or strong iron spoon to make a rather soft dough; as it cools, knead it a little with the hands, make the dough into small thin cakes or rolls; prick them to prevent blistering, and bake about twenty minutes in a hot oven. The baker—an iron one is best—should be well dusted with dry meal to prevent sticking.

The cakes should be one-third of an inch in thickness, and one and a half to two inches wide. When made into rolls (which is the best form, as it exposes the largest surface to the heat and forms a thinner and more tender crust,) they should be about the length and thickness of the finger.

When a large quantity is required, it is more convenient to make them diamond-shaped. The dough is rolled out, cut in slips an inch and a half or two inches wide, then cross-cut into diamond-shaped cakes. The knife, roller, and board should be kept well covered with dry meal.

Fine flour bread may be made light in the same way. But it must be mixed with *cold* instead of *hot* water. It requires baking from ten to fifteen minutes.

BATTER BREAD.—Mix wheat-meal with *cold* water to the consistence of ordinary batter for griddle cakes. Pour the batter into any convenient baking-dish—the bottom of which should be covered with meal to prevent sticking—and bake in a quick oven. The batter may be half an inch thick, or as thin as can be spread. The thinner it is the better, although if made very thin a large oven is required to bake much in quantity. For this reason the bread rolls are most convenient for families. An individual who makes bread only for number one, and who does not like the "muss" of working in dough, will find the batter-bread a very convenient article. I have, many a time, made it and had it cooking in a gas stove in less than two minutes from the time I commenced.

WHEAT-MEAL CRISPS.—Mix the meal with water, cold, warm, or hot, into a stiff dough; roll it out as thin as possible, and cut into small narrow pieces or strips, and bake in a quick oven. These are excellent for sour stomachs and irritable bowels.

WHEAT-MEAL CRACKERS.—These differ from the bread rolls in being very dry, hard, and brittle. In order to render them so, the dough is thoroughly kneaded, and then baked in a *brick* oven till the moisture is entirely evaporated. If kept dry they will retain their sweetness and rich flavor for several weeks. If kept in a very dry and very cool place they will remain good for several months. They are made a little smaller and a little thinner than the Boston cracker of the shops. All traveling invalids should supply themselves with these crackers. MILLER & BROWNING, No. 15 Laight Street, New York, manufacture them largely, and send them to order to any part of the country.

LOAF-BREAD.—Very good loaf-bread may be made of six parts of wheat-meal, two parts of corn-meal, and one part of mealy potatoes, mixed with boiling water, and baked in the ordinary way.

RYE-BREAD ROLLS.—Rye-meal [unbolted rye flour] may be made into bread rolls or batter-cakes in the same manner as for wheat-meal bread rolls. They are very light and delicious.

CORN-CAKE.—Wet coarse-ground Indian-meal with boiling water, roll it into a cake or cakes of half an inch in thickness, and bake in a hot oven. Some prefer this made with cold water, after the manner of the wheaten batter-bread. This is the old-fashioned and ever-to-be-admired "Jonathan-cake" —the "Johnny-cake" of "Down-East."

OAT-MEAL CAKES.—These may be made in the same manner as the wheaten bread rolls.

OAT-MEAL CRISPS.—Made in the same manner as the wheaten article. When these are thoroughly dried over a slow fire, they will, if kept in a dry place, remain good for months.

PUMPKIN BREAD.—Stewed and sifted pumpkin, or richly-flavored winter squash, may be mixed with meal of any kind, and made into bread or cakes, in any of the ways already mentioned.

FRUIT BREAD.—Stewed apples, pears, peaches, pitted cherries, black currants, or berries may be mixed with unbolted flour, and made into fruit bread. A little sugar added will convert the article into fruit cake.

SNOW BREAD.—When snow is plenty and clean, a light and beautiful article of bread can be made by adding to flour, or meal, two or three times its bulk of snow, and stirring them together with a strong spoon. It may be baked in the form of a cake or loaf an inch or two inches in thickness. The oven should be quite hot. It will bake in about twenty minutes. A little pulverized sugar, mixed with the flour or meal, will convert this bread into a very short and tender sweet-cake.

GRIDDLE CAKES.—Oat-meal, wheat-meal, or corn-meal may be made into a batter by mixing with cold water and baking on a soapstone griddle. Some prefer hot water for oat-meal.

SQUASH CAKES.—Mix flour or meal with half its bulk of stewed squash, or West-Indian pumpkin; add milk sufficient to make a batter and cook on a griddle.

PASTRY.—Baker's pastry, and also "home-made pies," as ordinarily manufactured, are among the worst of dietetic abominations. But pastry can be made so as to be not only a luxurious, but a wholesome article. Almost any kind of fruit, with a little sugar, and a crust of wheat-meal, or of rye and corn-meal, shortened with mealy potatoes, are all the materials required. Squash, pumpkin, and custard pies require the addition of milk.

PUDDINGS.—I regard all these dishes, even when made in the plainest manner possible, as things to be permitted rather than recommended to invalids. They are mushes, made thin, moistened, and baked. Indian-meal, hominy, rice, and wheaten grits are the best farinaceous articles for making puddings. Sago and barley are allowable. Stewed pumpkins, properly sweetened, with a small proportion of farina or corn-starch, with or without a little milk, makes a very simple and light dessert that some persons are very fond of.

MUSHES.—These are preferable to puddings. Wheaten grits and hominy, well boiled, are the best mushes. When wheaten grits are coarse-ground they require boiling five or six hours. For an ordinary family they may be ground in a large-sized coffee-mill; and if ground as fine as convenient, they will cook in an hour and a half. Rye-meal, Indian-meal, and oat-meal make favorite mushes also. Rice should be boiled fifteen to twenty minutes; avoid stirring it so as to break the kernels; turn off the water, and let it steam fifteen minutes. All mushes, when cold, may be cut into slices, and moderately browned in an oven, when they become as good as new—and even better.

2

GRUELS.—These are merely very thin mushes. They are properly regarded as "slop diet" for feeble invalids during convalescence after acute diseases, in cases of obstinate constipation, etc. Wheat-meal, corn-meal, rye-meal, and oat-meal are employed in gruel-making. About two tablespoonfuls of meal are mixed with a gill of *cold* water and the mixture is then stirred into a quart of boiling water, and boiled gently fifteen minutes. Rice gruel is useful in some cases of diarrhea.

PORRIDGES.—These are intermediate between mushes and gruels. Wheat-meal or oat-meal is usually employed. Half a pound of the meal to a little more than a quart of water is the usual proportion. They require boiling about twenty minutes. Raisins, pitted-cherries, black currants, or dried berries may be added if desired.

SOUPS.—Split-peas, beans, barley, and rice are employed in the preparations of hydropatic soups. One pint of split-peas, boiled for three hours, in three quarts of water, makes one of the best soups for vegetarians. Some add a trifle of sugar. Bean soup is made of similar proportions, and then boiled in a covered pan for four or five hours. Rice should be boiled until entirely soft. Barley should be soaked for several hours and then boiled slowly in a covered pan for four or five hours. Tomato soup, made in the following manner, is a pleasant and wholesome dish: Scald and peel good ripe tomatoes; stew them one hour, and strain through a coarse sieve; stir in a little wheaten flour to give it body, and brown sugar in the proportion of a teaspoonful to a quart of soup; boil five minutes. Okra, or gumbo, is a good addition to this and other soups.

BOILED GRAINS.—Wheat, rice, hulled corn, and samp, boiled until the kernels are entirely soft, but not broken nor dissolved, rank next to bread in wholesomeness. They may be eaten with syrup, sauce, sugar, milk or cream, or fruit.

APPLE DUMPLINGS.—Mix boiled mealy potatoes with flour into a dough; roll it out a little less than one-fourth of an inch in thickness; inclose in each dumpling a medium-sized apple, previously pared and cored, and boil or bake about an hour.

RICE APPLE PUDDING WITHOUT MILK.—Boil rice till nearly done, then stir in sliced tart apples, and cook about twenty minutes.

BOILED INDIAN PUDDING.—Wet coarse corn-meal with boiling water, add a little sugar or molasses, tie the pudding in a bag, leaving room for it to swell, and boil three or four hours.

APPLE JONATHAN.—Fill a baking-dish two-thirds full of sliced tart apples, sweeten to taste; mix wheat-meal with water and milk (a little cream will make the crust more tender) into a batter, and pour over the fruit until the dish is filled; bake until the crust is well browned.

RICH APPLE PUDDING.—Take equal quantities of very tart apples, well stewed and sweetened, and bread rolls or crackers, previously soaked soft in cold water; mix them and heat them thoroughly for a few minutes. Any tart fruit will answer in the above.

CRISPED POTATOES.—Boil good, sound mealy potatoes till a little more than half cooked; then peel them, and bake in a hot oven till moderately browned.

POTATO SHORTENING.—Pare and boil good mealy potatoes, choosing those which are of an even size; pour off the water, and sift, while hot, through a wire sieve. An equal quantity added to flour makes the best shortening in the world for bread, pastry, cakes, etc. A little cream added makes a richer but less wholesome article.

ANIMAL FOODS.—As I never recommend animal food to invalids, although I sometimes tolerate the use of it in special cases, my remarks under this head must be very limited.

Beef-steak, without butter or gravy, is perhaps the very best kind of flesh-food. Slightly corned beef, boiled until quite tender, is also admissible. Mutton chops, broiled, or the lean part of mutton, boiled, ranks next to fresh beef in wholesomeness. Eggs are not materially different in this respect. To cook them as hygienically as possible, pour boiling water on them, and let them remain on top of the stove, or near the fire, but not allowed to boil, for seven to ten minutes. Chicken, boiled or broiled, is next in order; and lastly, fish which are not oily, as cod, halibut, trout, perch, etc. Milk is rarely admissible. With dyspeptic, bilious, and rheumatic invalids it is decidedly objectionable. Nor should persons affected with constipated bowels, or profuse discharges of any kind, use it at all. Butter and cheese should be out of the question, although cream and curd may be allowed.

EXERCISE.

"LITTLE and often," is the rule for most invalids. All exercises should begin and end moderately. The kinds of exercises should be as varied as possible, so as to bring into action all the muscles of the system. Long walks should be alternated with frequent runs and occasional rests. The most severe exercises should be taken in the early part of the day. Those who are able should take moderately active exercise before bathing [except in case of the morning bath taken on first rising,] and still more active exercise immediately after each bath. A morning walk or ride before breakfast is always desirable. Calisthenic, gymnastic, and kinesipathic exercises and manipulations, except in their mildest forms, should only be taken when the stomach is nearly empty. Regularity is of great importance. Feeble invalids should commence all exercises very moderately, and gradually increase them in time and severity. Whenever much fatigued, rest or a change of exercise is advisable. Invalids should not get so fatigued as to be restless in consequence during the night, nor so much so that a night's rest will not remove all its disagreeable feelings. Those who can not go into the open air will derive great benefit from exercising in their rooms with the windows open. Dancing and dumb-bells are among the most convenient in-door exercises. As exercise develops strength, the weakest muscles should be exercised the most; but if very weak, *passive* exercises should be principally employed for a while, as rubbing, kneading, riding, sailing, etc. Invalids who do not react well after bathing, should be well rubbed over with a dry sheet by the hands of an attendant, and afterwards by the bare hands. Examples of all kinds of calisthenic and gymnastic exercises, illustrated with cuts, may be found in the author's "Family Gymnasium," published by FOWLER & WELLS, 389 Broadway, New York.

VENTILATION.

ALL persons generally, and invalids particularly, should be very careful in having an abundant supply of pure air. This is very apt to be neglected in sleeping apartments. In sitting-rooms, warmed by the hot-air stove or furnace, the air is rapidly contaminated unless special attention is paid to ventilation. Indeed, no room is fit to sit nor sleep in unless there is some inlet for the fresh air, and an outlet for the impure air. In fevers and other acute diseases, fresh air should in all weathers be freely admitted into the sick room; and in putrid, infectious, and contagious disorders, as yellow fever, small-pox, etc., the supply should be abundant. Invalids will find it an excellent practice to *ventilate* the lungs each morning before breakfast, by half a dozen or more deep inspirations and prolonged expirations.

LIGHT.

THE importance of light, as a remedial agent, is not sufficiently appreciated. Nearly all forms of disease are more severe and unmanageable in low, dark apartments. Many persons who live in elegant and expensively furnished houses so darken many of the rooms, in order to save the furniture, as to render the air in them very unwholesome. The scrofulous humors which prevail among those inhabitants of our cities who live in rear buildings and under-ground apartments, sufficiently attest the relation between sunshine and vitality. Invalids should seek the sunlight as do the flowers—care being taken to protect the head when the heat is excessive. Exposing the whole skin in a state of nudity, frequently, to the air, and even to the rays of the sun, is a very invigorating practice. For scrofulous persons this is particularly serviceable

CLOTHING.

THE physiological rule is, the less clothing the better, provided the body is kept comfortable. It should never be worn so tightly as to impede, in the least degree, the free motions of the body and limbs. Especially must it be loose and easy around the chest and hips, so as not to interfere with the action of the vital organs in respiration. Flannel garments next to the skin are objectionable. In very cold weather, thicker outside garments, or more of them, may be worn; but flannel under-shirts and drawers tend to make the skin weak and susceptible to colds. Invalids who are accustomed to them should leave them off in the spring or early part of the summer, and so invigorate the skin by bathing, etc., that they will feel no necessity for them the ensuing winter.

SLEEP.

INVALIDS generally do not sleep enough. The importance of sound, quiet, and sufficient sleep can not be too highly estimated, as may be inferred from the physiological fact, that it is during sleep that the structures are repaired. The materials of nutrition are digested and elaborated during the day; but assimilation—the formation of tissue—only takes place during sleep, when the external senses are in repose. Literary persons require more sleep, other circumstances being equal, than those who pursue manual-labor occupations. If the brain is not duly replenished, early decay, dementation, or insanity will result. The rule for invalids is, to retire early, and remain as long in bed as they can sleep quietly. If their dietetic and other habits are correct, this plan will soon determine the amount of sleep which they require. Gross, indigestible, and stimulating food, heavy or late suppers, etc., necessitate a longer time in bed, for the reason that the sleep is less sound. And for the same reason, nervine and stimulating beverages, as tea and coffee, prevent sound and refreshing sleep, and thus wear out the brain and nervous system prematurely. Those who are inclined to be restless, vapory, or dreaming, during the night, should not take supper.

BEDS AND BEDDING.

ALL bedding should be as *hard*, and all bed-clothing should be as *light*, as a due regard to comfort will permit. Feather beds are exceedingly debilitating. Hair, grass, husk, cork* shavings, straw, etc., mattresses, made soft and elastic, are the proper materials to sleep on in warm weather. In winter a light cotton mattress may also be employed.

---

* Cork shavings are a superior article, and their use is rapidly increasing. They may be had of MILLER & BROWNING, 15 Laight st., New York.

BODILY POSITIONS.

AVOID crooked bodily positions in walking, sitting, working, or sleeping. Always bend the body on the hip joints; never by crooking the trunk. Never lean forward while sitting so as to compress the stomach and lungs. Do not sleep on high pillows. Children are often injured and the spines distorted by this habit. Invalids who are so distorted, or so feeble that they can not keep the erect position in sitting but a few minutes at a time, should change their position frequently—walk, sit, and lie down, etc., so often as either position becomes painful.

NIGHT-WATCHING.

THE usual custom and manner of watching with the sick is very reprehensible. If any persons in the world need quiet and undisturbed repose, it is those who are laboring under fevers and other acute diseases. But with a light burning in the room, and one or more persons sitting by, and reading, talking, or whispering, this is impossible. The room should be darkened, and the attendant should quietly sit or lie in the same or in an adjoining room, so as to be within call, if anything is wanted. In an extreme case, the attendant can frequently step lightly to the bedside, to see that the patient is doing well; but all noise and all light should be excluded, except on emergencies. It is a common practice with watchers to awaken the patient whenever he inclines to sleep *too soundly*. But this is unnecessary, because when the respiration becomes very laborious, the patient will awaken spontaneously. Under the drug-medical dispensation the custom is to stuff the patient, night and day, with victuals, drink, or medicines, every hour or oftener, so that any considerable repose is out of the question. But, fortunately for mankind, the Hygienic system regards sleep as more valuable than the whole of them.

FRICTION.

FRICTION, more or less active, is desirable after all ordinary baths, except in cases of fevers and acute inflammations. And in some cases of tumors, enlarged joints, and torpid muscles, active and prolonged rubbing, in promoting absorption and increasing the circulation, greatly assists the curative process.

Many of the cures of these affections performed by specialists, in which cases thorough hand-rubbing is conjoined with the use of liniments, decoctions, and other medicamentums, are attributable mainly if not wholly to the friction employed. Wens, chronic swellings from sprains or bruises, etc., have been cured by the rubbing process.

ELECTRICITY.

THERE are two kinds of electrical force, mechanical and chemical. The former is the ordinary machine electricity, which operates mainly by producing shocks which agitate the motive fibers. It is quite analogous to friction in its effect, and is hence sometimes called friction-electricity. It is a convenient method for exercising, in many cases, particular sets of muscles, exciting action in some particular organ or part; and to this extent is a useful remedial agent.

GALVANISM.

THIS is generated by alternate layers of metallic plates of opposite electrical natures. It is a powerful chemical agent, and as such is extensively employed in the arts. Its chemical action enables it to effect, to some extent, the decomposition of foreign and effete matters in the fluids and tissues of

2*

the living system, and thus favor their elimination. The galvanic current will often excite action and sensibility in semi-paralyzed muscles and nerves, and is sometimes successfully resorted to for the purpose of allaying rheumatic and neuralgic pains. The galvanic battery in connection with the warm bath in the form of the electro-chemical bath, is probably the most convenient and efficient method of employing the galvanic influence as a depurating agent.

MAGNETISM.

WHATEVER may be the intrinsic nature of the mysterious property known as animal magnetism, and whatever may be its relation to the life-principle, it is certainly capable, under certain circumstances, of exercising a powerful influence over the vital functions. The salutary effects of a cheerful disposition, a hopeful mind and a healthy organism, upon the minds and bodies of invalids, are well known to physicians. Many persons are exceedingly susceptible to the influence of magnetism, while others can with great difficulty be impressed at all. In some cases it will quiet pain and restlessness, and produce sleep more effectually than opiates; and in rare cases it can be made an efficient anesthetic agent to suspend sensibility, so that surgical operations can be performed without pain. Its laws, however, are not yet sufficiently understood to enable us to reduce its remedial applications to any very definite rules.

CLEANLINESS.

FEW persons seem to have a proper idea of the full import of this term. Being next to godliness, the term, cleanliness, implies perfect purity in all our mental and organic relations. Many persons who are exceedingly nice and fastidiously neat in their attentions to the external skin, and in the matters of apparel, bedding, rooms, furniture, etc., are, notwithstanding, extremely heedless in regard to internal conditions and external surroundings. They will continually take into their stomachs and lungs such aliments and miasms as poison the blood and befoul the secretions; while they will permit the elements of contagion to accumulate to any extent in their cellars, yards, cesspools and out-buildings. I have known half a dozen members of a family to be prostrated with typhus fever, the chief cause being stagnant water and rotting vegetables in the cellar. Offal and garbage—dead and decomposing vegetable and animal matters of all kinds—in or around any dwelling, are a prolific source of disease. The hog-pen of many of our farmers causes more strange, putrid, and even fatal diseases than most persons suspect. I can hardly conceive of a fouler concentration of malignant and pestilent miasms than those which always emanate from a den of swine while undergoing the process of fattening. If folks will persist in keeping piggeries, they should be located so far from the dwelling-house that the abominable stench thereof will not be offensive to noses polite.

HYGIENIC HOME-TREATMENT:

OR

HAND-BOOK OF HYGIENIC PRACTICE.

ABORTION.—The expulsion of the fœtus before the seventh month is termed *abortion*; after the seventh month, *miscarriage*. The ordinary causes are violent exertion, intense mental emotion, plethora and constitutional frailty, acquired debility, dysmenorrhea, mechanical violence, drastic purgatives, powerful drugs, as quinine, tartar emetic, ergot. The chief danger results from hemorrhage or loss of blood. To prevent abortion, or to restrain the bleeding after it has occurred, the patient must be kept perfectly quiet in the horizontal position; cloths dipped in cold water applied to the lower abdomen; the feet must be kept warm; and in extreme cases it may be necessary to introduce a piece of soft sponge as nearly as possible to the mouths of the bleeding vessels.

ABSCESS.—A collection of purulent matter in a cavity, one of the results of inflammation. When practicable the pus should be evacuated, and the further extension of the inflammation prevented, and the part healed by tepid or cold applications, according to the degree of heat, and by strict attention to the general health.

ACATAPOSIS.—A term used sometimes for difficulty of swallowing, which affection may result from spasm of the muscles, or be caused by a thickening of the mucous membrane, or enlarged tonsils. When the affection is spasmodic, warm fomentations and warm hip-baths are indicated. In the other cases a plain and very abstemious diet, and a daily ablution, are the essentials of treatment. When the tonsils are very much enlarged and indurated it is sometimes necessary to remove them.

ACEPHALOCYST.—An Entozoa most frequently found in the liver, but sometimes in other organs and parts of the body. It is a hydatiform vesicle, without head or visible organs. The only assignable cause is gross alimentation, and the only remedy, a return to pure and simple food. But it happens unfortunately that their presence is seldom known except in post-mortem examinations.

ACHOLIA.—Deficiency or want of bile. See Liver Complaint.

ACHORES.—A term applied to *crusta lactea*, and also to small superficial ulcers of the skin. See Porrigo.

ACHYLOSIS.—Defective formation of Chyle. See Dyspepsia and Indigestion.

ACHYMOSIS.—Defective Chymification. See Indigestion.

ACMASTICUS.—A fever which preserves an equal intensity throughout its course. See Entonic Fever.

ACME.—The height of a febrile paroxysm.

ACNE.—A small pimple or tubercle on the face; or an eruption of distinct, hard, inflamed tubercles, usually appearing on the forehead, temples and chin. They are common to both sexes, but the most severe forms are seen in young men. Authors notice four varieties, the *simple, indurated, maggot pimple* and *rosacea*. Bad blood, gross food, torpid liver, and "nervous debility" are the common causes; and all the processes of purification and invigoration constitute the remedial plan. The Cosmetics, "Freckle eradicators" and "Skin beautifiers" of the quacks are worse than useless. I know many badly deformed faces which have entirely recovered after persevering in a life according to the laws of health for two or three years.

ACOSMIA.—A term applied to bald persons.

ACRASIA.—A term applied to intemperance or excess of any kind.

ACRATIA.—Impotence, weakness, fainting. See Syncope.

ACRIMONY.—An impure condition of the blood, resulting from retained bilious and other effete matters. The ancients, adopting the humoral pathology, conceived that an "acrimony of the humours" was the cause of many diseases. The moderns have unfortunately rejected this doctrine, and instead of seeking to eliminate the impurities, they counteract or subdue the remedial effort with narcotics, stimulants, alteratives, etc. The wet-sheet pack and the warm bath are the best detergent processes.

ACRODYNIA.—A term applied to a painful affection of the wrists and ankles especially, which appeared as an epidemic in Paris in 1828 and 1829. It was undoubtedly of a rheumatic nature, though some physicians imputed it to the vague phrase "Spinal irritation."

ACRORRHEUMA.—Rheumatism of the extremities.

ACROTISMUS.—See Asphyxia.

ACUTE.—Applied to disease this term means, rapid in progress and of short duration.

ADENITIS.—Glandular inflammation.

ADIPOSIS.—See Plethora.

ADYNAMIC.—A state of debility. Vital exhaustion. Low diathesis. Applied to fever, the word implies the atonic or typhoid form. Applied to inflammation, it means passive, in contradistinction to active.

AERIFLUXUS.—Flatulence, which see.

AERNO-ENTERECTASIA.—Tympanitis, which see.

AEROPHOBIA.—Dread of the air. This symptom frequently accompanies hydrophobia, hysteria and some other affections.

AEROTHORAX.—See Pneumothorax.

ÆTHERIZATION.—See Etherization.

AGUE.—See Intermittent Fever.

AGUE AND FEVER.—Intermittent Fever.

AGUE-CAKE.—A chronic enlargement of the liver or spleen—most commonly the spleen—which follows agues, and is distinctly felt by external examination. Nearly every person who has taken quinine frequently has some degree of this affection. It is to be remedied by the wet-girdle, hip-baths, a daily ablution, hot and cold foot-baths, and a rigidly abstemious diet. The Hydro-Electrical baths are admirable in these cases.

ALBUGINITIS.—A term applied to inflammations of the albumineous or white tissues. Some authors regard gout and rheumatism as species of albuginitis. See Arthritis.

ALBUMINURIA.—A disease of the urinary organs, characterized by the presence of albumen in the urine, and indicated by its coagulation on the application of adequate heat. It is generally attended with ulceration or fatty degeneration of the kidneys. It is justly regarded as a very dangerous disease; yet I have thus far succeeded in curing all the cases which I have treated hygienically, with a single exception. There is always a low grade of inflammation of the kidneys with a very inactive condition of the skin, and often a very torpid state of the liver. These conditions are attended with more or less pain, aching or distress in the region of the kidneys; much lameness or weakness in the small of the back, and lower extremities, coldness of the feet, and a variety of dyspeptic symptoms. The warm or vapor-bath, followed by the tepid ablution two or three times a week; the tepid or moderately warm hip-bath once or twice a day; the wet-girdle, whenever it can be worn without distress or chilliness, and the hot-and-cold foot-bath at bedtime, are the bathing processes to be resorted to. The diet should be restricted to unleavened bread, good fruit, and a small allowance of vegetables, and should be quite moderate in quantity. Water-drinking should be governed entirely by the thirst. The patient should indulge very moderately in active exercises, but passive exercises, as carriage riding, are highly useful.

ALBUMINURORRHEE.—Bright's disease of the kidney.

ALCOHOLISMUS.—A term recently applied by a writer in the Boston *Medical and Surgical Journal* to the alcoholic disease.

This subject is fully explained in the author's late work, "The True Temperance Platform."

ALOPECIA.—Baldness, falling off of the hair. The use of hot drinks, and the excessive use of common salt are frequent causes. Cut the hair short, wet the head morning and evening with cold water, and shampoo occasionally. Avoid "hair oils," "hair tonics," "hair invigorators," and hair humbugs generally.

AMAUROSIS.—Drop Serene, Gutta Serena, Black Cataract. Diminution or complete loss of vision, with no perceptible structural disorganization of the eye. It is usually imputed to a loss of power in the optic nerve; and this is generally caused by a viscid condition of the blood consequent on defective elimination of the effete matters. A torpid or inactive condition of the liver is almost always a prominent precedent condition. It may be induced suddenly by severe exposure to intense light, and is frequently induced by intemperance, gluttony, tobacco, excessive night study, etc. When the disease comes on gradually, letters and other objects seem misty, confounded, doubled, or intermixed, and sometimes undistinguishable. Insects, cobwebs and flashes of light often appear before the eye.

The malady is only curable in its incipient stage. The patient should at once adopt a rigidly simple and abstemious diet; sugar, butter, milk, and all "hydro-carbonaceous" articles must be avoided. If the external temperature is sufficient the wet-sheet pack should be employed daily; if not, the tepid half-bath, in the morning; the tepid hip-bath in the evening, and the hot-and-cold foot-bath at bedtime. I need hardly add that all exciting producing causes must be carefully avoided.

AMBLYOPIA.—The incipient stage of amaurosis.

AMENORRHŒA.—Obstruction of the menstrual or monthly flow. Of this affection there are two varieties. *Retention* and *Suppression*. *Retention of the Menses* may be caused by an imperforate hymen, or an obstruction of the uterine canal by viscid and concreted mucous, in which case the effused blood will be retained in the vagina, or in the cavity of the uterus. The symptoms which denote this affection are, an ædematous swelling of the feet and ankles at night, a swelling of the eyes and face in the morning, with more or less sense of weight or heaviness in the pelvic region. To be certain of the diagnosis it may be necessary to make a digital or instrumental examination.

When the cause of retention is an imperforate hymen, this can readily be obviated by a crucial incision, and when the os uteri or cervical canal are obstructed, warm water injections with the gentle use of the probe, or the application of a sponge tent, may be required.

Suppression of the menses is that form of Amenorrhœa in which the flux is arrested after having been once established. The chief constitutional symptoms are headache, palpitation, and difficult breathing. In many cases, complicated with dyspeptic conditions, there is a capricious appetite, and frequently a longing for such indigestible substances as clay, charcoal, slate-stone, etc. These patients are very liable to consumption.

The constitutional treatment is of vastly more importance than the local, though neither should be neglected. The bowels are usually constipated, and enemas should be employed daily until the fecal dejections become free and easy. The patient should exercise in the open air frequently, and as much as possible without great fatigue. Walking, riding, moderate dancing, and light gymnastics, are among the best exercises. Swedish Movements are especially beneficial to those who have contracted chests and weak abdominal muscles. The diet should consist mainly of coarse bread and fruit, with a moderate allowance of vegetables. Milk, butter, cheese, and sugar should be eschewed, nor should fine flour bread or puddings be used. Hip-baths, the wet-girdle, and foot-baths, of a temperature suited to the temperature of the patient, are always proper. In most cases one full bath per day is sufficient, and this may be the wet-sheet pack, or the warm bath followed by the tepid spray or sponge, or the tepid rubbing wet sheet, as may be found most agreeable to the patient. When there is much pain or distress about the loins or in the pelvic region, at the time for the menstrual discharge, the warm hip-bath or hot fomentations should be resorted to.

ANÆMATOSIS.—Defective preparation of the blood. See Anæmia.

ANÆMIA.—The opposite of Plethora; Exsanguinity, Bloodlessness. A state of the system in which the blood is deficient in quantity and especially deficient in the red corpuscles. The superficial capillaries are disproportionately bloodless, and there is every characteristic of debility. The treatment, in a general sense, consists in supplying the organism with whatever it can use under the circumstances. First in importance are air and exercise. Gentle bathing of the whole surface, with active, yet not violent friction, is in order. The diet should be very plain and limited in quantity to the capacity of the digestive organs. The patient should be careful to get sufficient sleep, and must, secondly, avoid all sources of mental disquietude. The "blood-food"—preparations of iron, hypophosphites, cod-liver oil, etc., which is almost invariably recommended by drug doctors in all cases of anæmia, is always pernicious, and not unfrequently fatally so.

ANÆSTHESIA.—Insensibility, privation of Sensation. It may be general or partial, and may be induced by all powerful narcotics, as chloroform, alcohol, opium, belladonna, and by some nervines, as sulphuric ether, and nitrous oxide. Electricity and magnetism will, with some persons, induce a state of insensibility, during which surgical operations may be performed without pain. Extreme cold, or congelation, renders the part to which it is applied insensible; it also diminishes and sometimes destroys the vitality of cancers and other morbid growths, which fact affords the rational basis of the refrigerating treatment of cancers and other tumors.

The remedy for anæsthesia is atmospheric air. In extreme cases the head should be moderately raised and inclined to one side, the tongue drawn forward so that it will not obstruct the glottis, and the patient exposed to a current of fresh air, or fanned vigorously.

ANAPHODISIA.—Absense of sexual desire. See Impotence and Sterility.

ANASARCA.—General Dropsy, Lucophleymatia. That form of dropsy in which the fluid is effused into the areolar or cellular tissue of the whole body. The swelling is first manifested around the ankles, and is characterised by tumefaction of the limbs, of the soft parts covering the abdomen, thorax, and even the face. The whole surface is dry, pale, and easily indented by pressure. When it supervenes upon chronic local disease, as consumption, albuminuria, lumbar abscess, hydrothorax, etc., it is generally fatal.

The proper plan of treatment contemplates the invigoration of the whole absorbent system, and the restoration of the cutaneous circulation. The diet should be light, dry, and largely frugivorous; the surface should be sponged daily with tepid water, and followed by active friction; the dry sheet rubbing should be employed once or twice a day. When the kidneys are very deficient in the excretion of urine, a warm-and-cool hip-bath should be taken daily, and the wet-girdle worn during the day, provided it does not cause chilliness, in which case it should be worn during the night. An important item in the dietetic treatment of dropsical patients, is that of eating *very slowly*, and this is still more important in the use of fruit. Half an hour is not too long a time in which to masticate and insalivate two good apples, or a pound of grapes.

ANCHYLOSIS.—See Ankylosis.

ANDROMANIA.—See Nymphomania.

ANEMIA.—See anæmia.

ANETUS.—Intermittent Fever, which see.

ANEURISM.—A tumor caused by the abnormal dilation of an artery, or of the heart. In *True Aneurism* the blood forms the tumor; and in *Spurious* or *False Aneurism*, the blood has escaped from the opened artery. There are three forms of the False Aneurism. 1, Diffused, which consists of an extravasation of the blood into the areolar texture of the part, immediately after the rupture or division of an artery. 2, *Circumscribed*, in which the blood issues from the vessel sometime after the receipt of the wound, and forms itself a sac in the neighboring areolar membrane. 3, *Aneurism by Anastomosis*, which arises from the simultaneous wounding of an artery and vein—the arterial blood passing into and producing a varicose state of the vein.

The treatment of aneurismal affections is mainly surgical, and consists in obliterating the dilated or communicating vessels, when practicable. But much may be done to prolong life, and in many cases, to prevent fatal consequences. It is obvious that all violent exertions which disturb the circulation will aggravate the malady; constipation of the bowels will, by obstructing the circulation, hasten an incurable condition or a fatal termination. The patient should be carefully regular in all personal habits; exercise moderately; diet temperately; and avoid all violent shocks, emotions, or agitations, of mind or body; and in all respects conform to organic law.

ANGEITIS.—A term applied to inflammation of vessels in general.

ANGINA.—The term is generic and is applied to a variety of affections of the throat and air passages, among which are *quinsy, croup, diptheria, laryngismus, laryngitis, aptha, pharyngitis, coryza, sternalgia,* etc., all of which will be treated of under their respective heads.

ANGINA PECTORIS.—This term is applied to an affection characterized by a violent pain about the sternum, or breast bone, extending towards the arms, accompanied with anxiety, difficult breathing, and a sense of suffocation. Some pathologists have regarded it as a *neuralgia of the heart*.

It may be relieved by hot fomentations to the chest, conjoined, in extreme cases, with warm sitz and foot-baths.

ANGINA PELLICULARIS.—See Croup and Diptheria.

ANGINA STRANGULATORIA.—This term is applied to inflammatory affections of the tonsils, glottis, windpipe, uvula, and palate, when attended with a sense of choking or strangling.

ANGINOSA.—Applied to that form of scarlet fever which is attended with swelling of the throat.

ANGINE.—See Globus Hystericus.

ANHÆMIA.—See Anæmia.

ANHELATION.—Short and rapid breathing. See Dyspnœa.

ANKYLOBLEPHARON.—A preternatural union between the free edges of the eyelids, the result of adhesive inflammation.

ANKYLOGLOSSIA.—Tongue-tied. It is caused by the shortness of the frænum, or an adhesion between its margins and the gums. In the former case the frænum may be divided with a pair of scissors, and in the latter the adhesion may be dissected away.

ANKYLOSIS.—Stiff-jointed. It is *complete* and *true* when there is a firm adhesion between the synovial surfaces, with union of the articular extremities of the bones, and *incomplete* or *false* when there is obscure motion.

The former condition is generally incurable. The latter may be greatly relieved, and often entirely cured, by fomentations, douches, persevering friction, while gently and gradually exercising the part.

ANOREXIA.—Want of appetite without loathing of food. It exists in the early state of most acute diseases, and is a symptom in many chronic diseases, particularly dyspepsia. The treatment should be directed to the primary malady, or to the constitutional condition.

ANOSMIA.—Loss of smell, a result of catarrh, the excessive use of snuff, opium, quinine, etc.

ANTEVERSION.—Displacement of the uterus, in which the body or fundus is directed forward toward the pubes and against the bladder, whilst the *os uteri* is turned backward toward the sacrum and lower bowel. To reposit the organ the fundus may be pushed upward with the finger, while the patient lies on the back with the hips well raised. When the organ and surrounding parts are feeble and relaxed, they must be invigorated by means of vaginal injections, hip-baths, abdominal manipulations, and all the appliances of the Hygienic System.

ANTHRACIA.—Carbuncular Exanthem. An eruption of imperfectly suppurating tumors, with indurated edges, generally with a foul, sanious core. They indicate a gross and putrescent condition of the body, and are always among the symptoms of *Plague* and *Yaws*. See Anthrax.

ANTHRACOSIS.—A species of carbuncle which affects the eyelids and globe of the eye. The term is also applied to the "black lung of coal miners," an affection induced by accumulation of carbonaceous particles in the lungs. Sometimes ulceration of the lungs results from this cause, and the malady is then termed *black phthisis*. See Melanosis.

ANTHRAX.—Malignant boil, carbuncle. An inflammation of the skin and areolar tissue, of a gangrenous tendency. It is frequently seen in the later stage of low fevers, and is sometimes among the critical manifestations of chronic diseases, in persons of impure blood or feeble vitality.

Carbuncles are also among the remote results of mercurial infection. Patients who have been salivated, or who have been subjected to the prolonged use of mercury in any form, are very liable to the most aggravated forms of malignant ulcers, which are very difficult to heal, as the bony structure is very liable to be involved in the disorganizing inflammation.

Keep the part constantly surrounded with wet cloths covered with dry, so long as there is any preternatural heat. Cavities should be filled, and abraded surfaces covered with flour, reapplied once a day; and when the edges of the ulcer become indurated or very painful, gentle douches with warm water, or mild fomentations, will relieve. I need hardly add that the general health must be properly attended to. The wet-sheet pack, warm baths, or the Hydro-Electrical baths should be employed to deterge mercurial and other impurities from the system, and salt, sugar, milk, butter, and cheese, must be excluded from the dietary.

ANEURESIS.—ANURIA. See Ischuria.

ANTIMONIALIS.—The antimonial disease, occasioned by tartar emetic and other preparations of antimony being administered as medicine, or accidentally taken into the system. The symptoms are, burning pain in the pit of the stomach, with retching or vomiting; purging; colicky pains; sense of tightness in the throat; and violent cramps. If the poison has been recently swallowed, an emetic of warm water should be taken; when small doses have been taken for days and weeks, the medicine must be got rid of through the excretory organs (the skin, liver, lungs, bowels, and kidneys). Pain and inflammation are to be allayed by fomentations and cold, wet cloths. The full warm bath is to be applied daily, followed by the tepid ablution.

ANTIGMATISM.—A term which has been lately applied to defective and indistinct vision, and which may be improved or remedied entirely by proper glasses. See Myopia.

ANTROVERSION.—See Anteversion.

ANXIETY.—Great restlessness and agitation with a distressing sense of oppression at the epigastrium. It is a prominent symptom in the early stage of all malignant fevers, and of many acute diseases, and may attend the latter stage of all. It is also induced by overloading the stomach, and by taking indigestible substances. It may be relieved by warm water drinking and fomentations. When excessive or indigestible aliment is the cause, a warm-water emetic is the remedy.

AORTITIS.—Inflammation of the aorta, and, in my opinion, a nosological mistake.

APATHY.—Suspension or loss of the moral emotions. It takes place in malignant fevers, and in some chronic diseases attended with extreme congestion of the brain. I have had several patients who evinced no desire to live, and who did not seem to care what happened to themselves or to others. Fortunately the symptom is only temporary, and disappears entirely on a removal of the cause.

APEPSIA.—See Dyspepsia.

APHONIA.—Loss of voice. Aphonia often exists as a symptom in catarrh. It is sometimes caused by paralysis of some part of the vocal apparatus, but is more frequently the consequence of debility or extreme relaxation of the respiratory muscles. In some cases it has resulted from a misuse of the respiratory muscles, by which the effort of phoriation is thrown on the wrong muscles. Strong mental emotions are sometimes the cause of this affection.

The remedial measures must of course have reference to the causes. Whatever will improve the whole breathing apparatus, will conduce to the recovery of the voice. In cases of general debility, or of abuse or misuse of the vocal organs, vocal gymnastics are especially serviceable; but great care should be taken to have the dorsal and abdominal muscles called into play, or the exercises will be worse than useless.

APHRONIA.—A synonym for Apoplexy, which see.

APHROSYNE.—Delirium, Insanity.

APHTHÆ.—Thrush or sore mouth, stomatitis. There are two varieties, the *common, white,* or *milk thrush,* and the *black* or *malignant.* Both forms, are symptomatic of bad digestion or impure blood. Hot drinks, strong green tea, strong cheese, and stale butter and meats sometimes induce the mild form of the affection in adults. When it affects nursing infants, the mother should regulate her diet properly, and the mouth of the child be frequently wet with a teaspoonful of cold water. The malignant form is frequently an accompaniment of putrid fevers, and is always to be treated with the constitutional processes of purification—the warm bath, the wet-sheet pack, or frequent ablutions, as the temperature of the patient indicates. In all cases, cold applications to the throat, with bits of ice or sips of cold water taken into the mouth frequently, are the proper local measures.

APNEUSTIA.—Apnœa, Asphyxia.

APNŒA.—Insensible respiration, Orthopnœa. See Asphyxia.

APONEUROSITIS.—Inflammation of an aponeurosis. Apply very cold wet cloths until relieved.

APOPLEXY.—This disease is characterized by a loss of consciousness, sensibility, and voluntary motion. It is usually attended with more or less rigidity of the limbs, with puffy, stertorous breathing. Authors distinguish two species, the *Sanguineous*, and the *Serous*, as the surface is flushed or pale. The immediate cause is congestion or compression of the brain. The remote causes are whatever obstructs the circulation, or renders the blood thick and viscid. Plethoric persons are peculiarly subject to the disease. Excessive alimentation is its most common cause:

Place the patient in an easy position with the head well raised. Free the bowels with an enema of tepid water. If the breathing is very laborious, apply fomentations to the abdomen. Apply hot bottles to the feet, if there is the least indication to chilliness; wet cloths should be applied to the head. When the surface is warm and feverish, it should be sponged two or three times a day with tepid water, followed by gentle friction.

APOSTEMA.—The word is sometimes applied to tumors in general, but is usually employed as a synonym of Abscess, which see.

APYREXIA.—The state of the system (DUNGLISON says it is the *condition* of an intermittent fever), between the paroxysms of an intermittent fever. The term is sometimes applied to the non-febrile period of other acute diseases. Strictly, it means the absence of the hot stage of a febrile disease.

ARACHNITIS.—Inflammation of the arachnoid membrane of the brain. See Copalitis.

ARANEA.—See Tarentula.

ARDENT FEVER.—Synocha, or Inflammatory Fever.

ARDOR URINÆ.—A scalding sensation experienced while the urine is passing over the inflamed mucous membrane of the urethra, or neck of the bladder. It is a symptom of gonorrhœa and leucorrhœa, and may be induced by acrid poisons, as turpentine, cantharides, etc. The constant application of tepid, cool, or cold water, is necessary until relieved.

ARENOSA URINA.—Sandy Urine. See Gravel.

ARGEMA.—A white spot, or ulceration of the eye. See Leucoma.

ARGENTITIS.—I have introduced this term for the malady known as the *Blue Disease,* and which is caused by nitrate of silver (*argenti nitras*) administered as a medicine. Such cases are not so frequent as formerly, for the reason that the drug is less used. The malady has thus far proved incurable. A few years ago, when the Electro-Chemical baths were first introduced in this city, it was claimed that they were capable of removing this discoloration. And an individual who was frequently seen in the streets, and who had been employed for years to hand out the programmes in front of the American Museum, was reported to have been cured. And what is singular, one operator in this city and another in Philadelphia, each claimed to have cured him. But, as it happened, the blue-dyed patient continued to present the same external appearance.

ARGYRIA.—A term applied to the discoloration of the skin, occasioned by the internal use of lunar caustic, or nitrate of silver.

ARNICALIS.—A term I have taken the liberty to apply to the disease or "medicinal effects" occasioned by the drug Arnica

Montana. The symptoms are—stupor, dilated pupil, anxiety, spasmodic actions of the muscles, and in extreme cases, coma, involuntary evacuations and paralysis. The patient should be kept quiet, with the head well raised, as in apoplexy, and freely exposed to the fresh air. Cold applications to the head and warm applications to the feet will assist the recovery. When the skin is preternaturally warm, it should be sponged with tepid water.

ARSENICALIS.—This term has already been employed by some nosologists to indicate arsenical disease. It is characterized by a burning heat in the stomach. Some degree of coppery or metallic taste in the mouth, with fleecy or spongy gums, and a swelling, fullness or puffiness of the face. To eliminate the poison the vapor bath, wet-sheet pack, and Hydro-Electrical bath are useful. I have no faith in chemical antidotes. They are proper when the drug is in the stomach, but when it is diffused throughout the system they are worse than useless.

ARSENICISMUS.—Poisoning by arsenic.

ARTERITIS.—Inflammation of an artery. Says Professor GILMAN, of the New York College of Physicians and Surgeons: "The continued application of cold water has more power to prevent inflammation than any other remedy." He should have said, to *cure* inflammation. Cold water may either prevent inflammation, or cause it, according to the circumstances of the case and the mode of its application.

ARTHRAGRA.—See Gout.

ARTHRITIS.—This term is usually employed generically to comprehend all forms of gout and rheumatism.

ANTHROCHONDRITIS.—Inflammation of the cartilages and joints. Apply cold water.

ARTHRODYNIA.—Pain in the joints. It is usually of a rheumatic or mercurial origin. Foment the part and then apply the wet bandage.

ARTHROSIA.—This is a generic term applied to painful inflammatory swellings of the joints. It induces many forms of gout and rheumatism.

Arthropongus.—A white, fungous tumor of the joints. It may be removed by congelation, or caustic, or both.

Asbestos Scall.—See Eczema of the Hairy Scalp.

Ascaris—Ascarides.—Thread, Pin, or Maw Worms. Characterized by a long, cylindrical body, extenuated at the extremities. There are supposed to be several species of entozoa included in the genus Ascaris. Copious enemas of pure water, and a dietary of coarse bread and fruit, with unseasoned vegetables, will in due time destroy them by obviating the cause on which their existence depends. Sugar, all greasy substances, and fermented breads, should be abstained from by all who are troubled with worms.

Ascites.—Hydrops Abdominis, (Dropsy of the Belly.) A collection of watery fluid in the abdomen. Characterized by increased size of the abdomen, fluctuation, and the usual signs of serous accumulation. Ascites proper is dropsy of the peritoneum, or lining membrane of the abdomen. When the constitutional vigor is not greatly reduced, it may be removed by absoption, or by tapping—*paracentesis.* When the fluid is saccated (collected in separate cysts) it is incurable. In some cases the watery accumulation is exterior to the peritoneum.

The warm wet-sheet pack, or the alternate warm and tepid rubbing sheet, with a dry and abstemious dietary, are the most effectual measures of treatment.

Asphyxia.—Pulselessness, Acrotismus, Apparent Death, Suspended Animation. The immediate cause is the non-conversion of venous into arterial blood; or, in other words, the retention of effete carbonaceous matter. The exciting causes are the presence of irrespirable gases, or the absence of atmospheric air, as in the cases of hanging and drowning. Narcotic fumes, and noxious vapors of various kinds, will induce it. The "choke-damp," or carbonic acid gas, which accumulates in deep caves, or in the bottom of dry wells, is one of the most frequent causes of death of Asphyxia. Chloroform, ether and other anesthetic agents, when administered without due precautions, sometimes induce the asphyxiated state, ending in death.

Atmospheric air is the only remedy. The patient should be placed in a current of fresh air, or fanned vigorously, and the tongue drawn forward. This last point is exceedingly important, and lives have been lost by not properly attending to it. The tongue is paralyzed and lies like a dead mechanical weight in the back part of the mouth, closing the glottis and completely excluding the atmospheric air from the lungs. To favor the inclination of the tongue forward, the patient should be turned on one side with the face inclining downward.

When the patient has been for a long time exposed to mephitic gases or vapors, or submerged, the restoration of the respiratory function can often be achieved as follows: Support the patient in a sitting posture, carry the arms gradually upward and outward above the head, and then as gradually depress them downward and forward, the whole to be performed sixteen to eighteen times per minute; during the downward motion an attendant should press firmly against the abdominal muscles. The object is to imitate the respiratory motions as nearly as possible, by which means a sufficient quantity of air may be made to enter the lungs to reinvigorate the circulation of the blood, and set the whole machinery of life in motion again.

The strangling is not occasioned, as is commonly supposed, by the water or noxious gases or vapors entering the lungs, but by the spasmodic closure of the glottis to keep them out.

ASSULTUS.—Attack. When physicians learn that diseases are not things, or entities, foreign to the living organism, but that they are, on the contrary, the actions of the vital powers in self-defence, we shall hear no more of diseases "attacking" us, "running through" us, "becoming seated" within us, being "self-limited," "deriving laws from their nature," etc., etc.; nor will physicians then think of "breaking up," or "neutralizing" or "counteracting," or "suppressing," or "subduing" disease, as is now the fashion. They will only seek to regulate and direct the remedial action, and supply the living system with whatever of normal (not morbific) agents it can use under the circumstances.

ASTHENIA.—*Vis Imminuta.* Applied by BROWN to designate debility of the whole system, in contradistinction to *Stenia,* the state of augmented vitality. The Brunonian hypothesis is very absurd in theory, and very disastrous in practice.

ASTHENOPIA—WEAK-SIGHTEDNESS. Ascertain and remove the cause.

ASTHMA.—There are many varieties of asthmatic affections, but the principal are the *Common,* or *Spitting*—Asthma Humidum; the Dry—*Asthma Siccum,* and the *Hay,* or *Harvest,* or *Fever* Asthma. The first variety is attended with copious expectorations; in the second variety the expectoration is scanty; the third variety appears in the haying or harvest season only. A kind of asthma, called *Grinders,* or *Grinder's Rot,* is sometimes caused by the inhalation of earthy and metallic particles, and affects stone-cutters and metallic instrument-grinders. More frequently, however, the disease is manifested in some one of the several forms of consumption.

The immediate cause of asthmatic respiration is, in a great majority of cases, an enlarged or congested state of the liver; noxious particles received into the lungs, repelled eruptions, suppressed discharges, rank odors, damp weather, dietetic errors, and strong mental emotions, are frequent exciting causes.

When the temperature of the patient will admit, the wet-sheet pack should be the leading bath, repeated daily, or every other day. When the temperature is lower, the tepid half-bath, followed by the pail douche, should be taken daily. The wet girdle should be worn about one-half of the time, and a moderately cool hip-bath taken once or twice a day, for ten or fifteen minutes. Feeble patients should take the hot and cold foot-bath at bed-time. Fomentations to the abdomen may be resorted to for temporary alleviation during the paroxysm.

The dietary can hardly be too strict, and must be very abstemious. Milk is objectionable, and recovery will be accelerated, if every kind of animal food is abstained from.

ATHEROMA.—A tumor formed of a cyst containing a pulpy or fatty matter, like pap. It can best be removed with the knife.

ATONY.—Want of tone. General Debility. *Atonic* is, and properly, applied to all chronic diseases, and to all fevers, except the inflammatory.

ATRABILIS.—Black Bile, or Melancholy. The ancient physicians ascribed many cases of hypochondriasis, mania, melancholy, etc., to the predominance of black bile; but there does not happen to be any such humor. Torpidity of the liver is a common cause of those affections.

ATROPHY.—Wasting of the Body, Marasmus. A condition which may more or less attend any disease.

AURA.—The sensation of a vapor rising from the body or limbs to the head or throat, and inducing a feeling of suffocation. It sometimes precedes paroxysms of epilepsy and hysteria, and has been termed *Aura Epileptica* and *Aura Hysterica.*

AURIUMALIS.—The effects of the medicinal preparations of gold (*Aurum*) are very similar to those of mercury. They have been employed experimentally as substitutes for the mercurials in scrofulous and syphillitic diseases, and in various cachexias. The gold malady is to be treated like all other mineral poisons, with all the eliminating appliances of the Hygienic system.

AUTUMNAL FEVER.—Remittent and intermittent fevers occur most frequently in the fall of the year, and are termed *Autumnal.* The remittent type is often termed *Bilious Fever.*

BALANITIS, BALANORRHŒA.—Spurious Gonorrhœa. A mucous or muco-purulent discharge from the urethra without venereal infection. For the treatment, see Leucorrhœa and Gleet.

BALBUTIES.—Traulismus, Stammering, St. Vitus' Dance of the Voice. The term is also applied to a vicious and incomplete pronunciation, in which almost all of the consonants are replaced by the letters B and L. Apply to a good elocutionist.

BARBRIERS.—*Beriberi.* A paralytic affection prevalent in India. The subjects of the disease are mostly persons of weakly constitutions and dissipated habits, and the termination is usually fatal. These circumstances sufficiently suggest the remedial plan.

BARRENNESS.—See Sterility.

BELCHING.—See Eructation.

BELLADONNALIS.—I venture to designate by this term the disease which is the aggregate of the poisonous effects of the *medicine* known as Atropa Belladonna, or deadly night-shade. The symptoms are stupor, numbness, dizziness, dimness of vision, nausea, dilated pupil, delirium, and, in extreme cases, convulsions. The treatment is the same as for Arnicalis.

BELLY-ACH.—See Colic.

BENIGN.—Diseases of a mild character are so termed.

BERIBERI.—See Barbiers.

BEX—See Cough.

BEZOAR.—A calculous concretion found in the stomach, intestines, and bladder of animals. They were primarily regarded as possessing wonderful medicinal virtues. Urinary calculi were once employed as powerful alexipharmics, or antidotes. Biliary and lachrynal calculi have also been employed in medicine. The Bezoard of the Indian Porcupine was formerly sold at an enormous price in Spain and Portugal.

BILIOUS, BILIOUSNESS.—This term is applied somewhat loosely to various diseases, and to many conditions of the system in which there is an exaction of biliary matter, inordinate in quantity or acrid and irritating in quality. It is sometimes employed in a very different and even in the very opposite sense, to denote a condition of torpor or inactivity of the liver, in which the biliary elements remain in the blood, or are partially expelled through the other enunctories, as in jaundice, and a variety of cutaneous disorders. The phrase " bilious attack," is applied to the disarrangement or disturbance of the digestive organs, consequent on the presence of morbid bile. Some fevers are termed " bilious," as are

HAND-BOOK OF HYGIENIC PRACTICE.   **BON.**

some forms of visceral inflammation, because of the free excretion of bile which attends their early stage. A variety of humors, eruptions, and nameless skin diseases, as well as many apthous, diptheretic, and cankerous conditions of the mucous membranes, are attributable, more than to any single cause, to a defective action of the liver. They are so many manifestations of "biliousness."

To remedy all of these conditions, a plain, simple dietary, with general bathing, according to the circumstances of the disease and the condition of the patient, are indispensable. The indications of cure are, to purify the mass of blood of its biliary elements, and to restore the function of the liver.

BISMUTHITIS.—I do not find this term in the Medical Lexicon, but I apply it to the bismuth disease, caused by the medicinal administration of the subnitrate of bismuth. The symptoms are, great heat or sense of burning in the stomach, thirst, furred tongue, vertigo, syncope, etc. The remedy is negative—let the drug alone.

BLACK DEATH.—This term was applied to the plague during its prevalence in the middle ages.

BLACK LUNG.—See Anthracosis.

BLACK TONGUE.—A term which has been applied to Putrid Sore Throat, which see.

BLEB.—See Bulla.

BLENNORRHAGIA, BLENNORRHŒA.—See Gonorrhœa.

BLEPHAROPTHALMIA, BLEPHAROPTHALMITIS.—See Opthalmia.

BLEPHAROPTOSIS.—A falling down of the upper eye-lid over the eye. It is an indication of great congestion of the brain, and often one of the precursors of apoplexy or palsy.

BLUE DISEASE.—Cholera, Spasmodic, which see.

BOIL.—See Turunculus.

BONA FEVER.—A malignant fever which prevailed amongst the troops of the garrison at Bona, in Algeria, from 1832 to

1835, has been so called. It did not differ in any essential particular from the ordinary typhus fever of camps and hospitals.

BONE FEVER.—Inflammation of the Bone.

BONES, BRITTLENESS OF THE.—See Fragilitas Ossium, and Mollities Ossium.

BORBORYGMUS.—The noise made by flatus or gas in the intestines. Any condition of indigestion which favors the fermentation of the food, tends to the production of flatulence. Sips of warm water will relieve it, and a proper dietary may cure.

BOTHRIOCEPHALUS.—Broad Tape-Worm. See Tænia.

BOULIMIA.—Insatiable hunger. It sometimes affects hysterical patients, and pregnant women. Dyspeptics are often troubled with an insatiate appetite or craving. The remedy is dry, solid food, which compels the patient to masticate very slowly, as hard crackers, parched corn, and, for those who have good teeth, raw wheat.

BOURGEONS.—See Gutta Rosea.

BRADYSURIA.—See Dysuria.

BRASH, WATER.—See Pyrosis.

BRASH, WEANING.—A severe diarrhœa occurring at the time of weaning. The warm-bath morning and evening, and proper attention to diet, are the remedial measures.

BREAST, ABSCESS OF.—Milk Abscess, Mammary Abscess. See Mastodynia Apostematosa.

BREAST-PANG.—See Angina Pectoris.

BREATH, OFFENSIVE.—This depends on decaying teeth, impure blood, foul secretions and filthy habits, as tobacco-using, liquor-drinking, pork-eating, etc. Probably constipated bowels is the immediate cause of more feted and offensive breaths than all other causes combined.

BRIGHT'S DISEASE OF THE KIDNEY.—A granular disease of the cortical part of the kidney which gives occasion to the excretion of urine that contains albumen; so named, because it was first described by Dr. BRIGHT. See Albuminuria.

BROKEN-WINDEDNESS.—Asthma.

BROMIDROSIS.—A term applied to offensive sweat. The causes and cure are indicated under the head of Breath, Offensive.

BRONCHITIS.—Inflammation of the lining, or mucous membrane of the bronchial tubes. It has been called Pulmonary Catarrh, Angina Bronchialis, Humid Pleurisy, etc. Laryngitis and Follicular Inflammation of the Throat, and even chronic Tonsilitis, are often miscalled Bronchitis, and all indiscriminately treated with the murderous fumigations, inhalations, and cauterizations of poisonous drugs. *Acute Bronchitis* is attended with fever, and requires precisely the same treatment as inflammation of the lungs. See Pneumonia. *Chronic Bronchitis* is one of the forms of consumption, and requires all the Hygienic appliances applicable to that disease.

In the early stages, the chest wrapper should be worn constantly, and derivative baths frequently employed. The tepid hip-bath, and hot-and-cold foot bath should be taken once or twice daily, and a full tepid or warm bath daily, each other day, semi-weekly or weekly, according to the patient's reactive power. The diet must be very simple and rather abstemious, and the patient should exercise in the open air all he possibly can, without great fatigue. Tobacco-users, who have chronic bronchitis, must renounce the luxury or expect to die.

In the early stages, the wet-sheet pack may be advantageously employed, daily or tri-weekly; and in all cases, the "Swedish movements" are admirable.

Bronchitis may be distinguished from laryngitis and "throat-ail" by the pain and tenderness being deep-seated and diffused in the chest; and chronic bronchitis may be distinguished from pleurisy or pneumonia by the absence of fever of the continued type.

BRONCHOCELE.—Swelled Neck, Goitre. An enlargement of the thyroid gland, sometimes amounting to a very large tumor, and seriously obstructing respiration. It is usually curable in its early stages, and but rarely afterwards. The patient must avoid hard water, drink only soft and pure water, and only so much as actual thirst demands; restrict the diet to plain, solid food, and be abstemious in quantity. Cold wet cloths should be worn around the neck, and a moderate douche, if practicable, applied two or three times a day. If the patient is in otherwise good health, the wet-sheet pack for an hour daily, followed by a moderate douche along the spine, will assist the absorption of the tumor. But if the general circulation is feeble, the tepid rubbing sheet should be preferred. Gentle and persevering friction to the tumor will often assist in its removal.

BRONCHOCEPHALITIS.—Hooping-Cough. See Pertussis.

BRONCHORRHŒA.—An increased excretion of mucus from the air passages. It is symptomatic of catarrh, indigestion, and various other maladies.

BRUISE.—Contusion. If there is heat with swelling, apply cold water; if not, foment the part or apply warm water, and then apply cold wet bandages.

BRYGMA.—Grinding of the teeth. A common symptom of teething in children, and of gastric irritation in both children and adults.

BUBO.—An inflammatory swelling of the glands of the groin. The term is sometimes applied also to a similar affection of the glands of the axilla or armpit. There are three varieties of this disease: 1. Simple, not connected with infection. 2. Venereal, occasioned by the venereal virus. 3. Pestilential, an accompaniment of the plague.

In each of these cases, the primary or constitutional condition must be attended to. The local treatment consists of frequent tepid or cool hip-baths, and the constant application of cold wet cloths. When the swelling is attended with throbbing pain, indicative of suppuration, warm water should be applied and the full warm-bath taken once or twice a day; or, if this is impracticable, the warm sitz-bath will answer very well.

BUBONALGIA.—Pain in the groin. It may be neuralgic or inflammatory. In the former case apply hot fomentations; in the latter, cold wet cloths.

BUBONOCELE.—Rupture of the groin, Inguinal Hernia. It may be relieved by a well-adjusted truss, and is sometimes cured by a surgical process.

BUCKET FEVER.—Dengue, which see.

BUCNEMIA.—See Elephantiasis.

BUFF, INFLAMMATORY, BUFFY COAT.—Corium Phlogisticum. A state of the blood in which, in consequence of disease, the fibrinous element, instead of being assimilated, remains in the blood and undergoes more or less alteration. The rational remedy is to remove the cause of the disease; but physicians have, most absurdly, for several thousands of years, been in the habit of taking the blood out by opening a vein with a lancet. How this is to remedy the difficulty, no advocate of venesection has ever told us, and probably never will.

BUGANTIA.—See Chilblain.

BULLA.—A Blob. A portion of the cuticle detached from the skin by the interposition of a transparent, watery fluid. It is the consequence of biliary obstruction of some morbid humor or impurity of the blood, and may be cured by means of frequent tepid ablutions, and a plain, simple diet. When it occupies a large surface, the wet-sheet pack should be employed.

BUNIOID.—A term applied to a cancer which bears some resemblance to a turnip.

BUNION, BUNYON.—An enlargement with inflammation of the bursa mucasa at the inside of the ball of the great toe. Alternate hot and cold foot-baths, with due attention to the general health, will remove or relieve them.

BURN.—An injury caused by extreme heat. In no diseases are there greater discrepancies of treatment by the drug doctors, than in burns and scalds. Some recommend the stimulating, and others the opposite, or antiphlogistic plan; while the specifics recommended by regular and irregular physicians are innumerable. The reason of this confusion worse confounded is, that the great majority of the cases will recover more or less perfectly with or without almost any treatment, and in spite of much mal-medication.

The principle of treatment is, to regulate the temperature of the part, and protect abraded surfaces from the contact of atmospheric air. When the injury is not deep, the application of flour alone will soon relieve the pain, and, if promptly applied, may prevent blistering, or the destruction of the cuticle. When the injury is deeper, the part should be held in cool water, of a temperature most agreeable to the patient, or cold wet cloths may be applied, and frequently changed. Should the cuticle or parts beneath slough off, the exposed surface should be kept constantly covered with dry flour, over which cold wet cloths may be applied.

BURNING OF THE FEET.—Persons of feeble circulation and of a bilious condition of the blood, are liable to this sensation, which is readily relieved by hot and cold foot-baths. In a singular cachectic disease, which occurs in India, the most prominent symptom is a sense of burning in the feet.

CACHECTIC.—Pertaining to a morbid condition of the system. A person affected with cachexia.

CACHEXIA, CACHEXY.—A bad habit, or depraved condition of the body, as in scrofula, scurvy, cancerous and venereal diseases, dropsies, etc.

CACHINNATIO.—A tendency to immoderate laughter, as in hysterical and maniacal affections.

CACODÆMON.—An evil spirit, to which were ascribed many disorders. Nightmare. See Incubus.

CALCULI.—Concretions of excrete or earthy matters which may form in any part of the body, but are most frequently found in the organs that serve as reservoirs, and in the excretory ducts and canals. They have been met with in the tonsils, joints, biliary ducts, intestines, lachrymal ducts, mammary glands, pancreas, pineal gland, prostate gland, lungs, salivary, spermatic and urinary passages, and in the uterus. The causes are, an excess of earthy, saline, or alkaline particles taken with the food, the use of mineral waters, the drinking of hard water, chalk, lime, magnesia, etc., taken as medicines.

The general remedial plan consists in the avoidance of the causes, and the use of such measures as will deterge the system of all existing impurities. A strict dietary, with a daily ablution or pack, and free but not excessive water-drinking, are the essentials.

CALCULI, ARTHRITIC.—Nodes, Chalk-Stones, Concretions which form in the ligaments and within the capsules of the joints of persons affected with the gout. Their composition is, soda, uric acid, and a little animal matter. In some instances, urate of lime and chloride of sodium are present also. A persevering Hygienic regimen will often remove every vestige of these concretions.

CALCULI, BILIARY.—Gall-Stones, Chololithus, Biliary Concretions. In some cases these concretions are only the elements of bile thickened; some contain *Picromel;* and the majority are composed of a small quantity of the yellow matter of the bile, with a large proportion of *Cholesterin.* They are most frequently found in the gall-bladder, but sometimes in the substance of the liver, in the branches of the *hepatic duct,* and in the common duct of the liver, and gall-bladder, (*Ductus Communis Choledochus*). Their presence does not always cause much uneasiness, but sometimes they occasion abscess and biliary fistulæ. The passage of gall-stones is very painful, often excruciatingly so, and can only be relieved by copious warm water drinking, hot fomentations to the abdomen, and warm hip-baths.

CALCULI, OF THE EAR.—These are merely indurated cerumen, and are a frequent cause of deafness. They can be easily seen, and may be removed with forceps, after being detached by repeated injections of warm water.

CALCULI, LACHRYMAL.—Concretions in the lachrymal passages sometimes cause abscesses and fistulæ; which cannot be healed until they are removed.

CALCULI, OF THE MAMMÆ.—These concretions are rare, but have been found in abscesses of that organ.

CALCULI, OF THE PANCREAS.—These are not detected during life, hence little is known of them.

CALCULI, OF THE PINEAL GLAND.—Their composition is phosphate of lime, but no symptoms indicate their presence during life.

CALCULI, OF THE PROSTATE GLAND.—These are generally composed of phosphate of lime. They occasion a sense of weight or heaviness, and more or less disturbance in urination.

CALCULI, PULMONARY.—Consumptives often expectorate concretions formed of carbonate of lime and a little animal matter.

CALCULI, SALIVARY.—Concretions in the salivary glands, or in their excretory ducts, are usually composed of phosphate of lime and animal matter.

CALCULI, SPERMATIC.—These cannot be detected during life, but are sometimes found after death, in the vesiculæ seminales. Their constitutents are unknown.

CALCULI, OF THE STOMACH AND INTESTINES.—Enterolithus. Calculi in the stomach are rare; in the intestines they are more frequently met with; almost any foreign substance may supply a nucleus. They are ordinarily found between the valves of the small intestines, or in the cells of the large. Sometimes they form a movable tumor which may be felt through the walls of the abdomen. A plain, unconstipating diet, with occasional copious enemas, and judicious manipulations of the abdomen—rubbing, kneading, etc.—will cause them to be evacuated in due time.

CALCULI, OF THE TONSILS.—These are readily recognized both by the sight and touch.

CALCULI, URINARY.—Several varieties of concretions are formed of the crystallizable substances in the urine. Their chief components are, Lithic Acid, Phosphate of Lime, Ammoniaco-Magnesian Phosphate, Oxalate of Lime, Cystic Oxide, and Xanthic Oxide.

Concretions formed in the kidneys, called *Renal* Calculi, have generally a very irregular shape, and often cause intense pain while being expelled, attended sometimes with inflammation, and turbid or bloody urine. Warm water, externally and internally, affords all the relief possible.

CALCULI, VESICAL.—Stone in the Bladder. These are indicated by a sense of weight in the perineum, and often a sense of a body moving or rolling when the patient changes position; pain or itching at the extremity of the urethra; frequent desire to urinate; sudden interruption of the stream; and occasionally bloody urine. But assurance should always be rendered doubly sure by an examination with the sound. In some cases they will be entirely dissolved and pass away, in consequence of a rigidly *antilithic* regimen. In other cases they can be broken into fragments in the bladder—*Lithotrity* —so as to pass out through the urethra with the urine. But in many cases they can only be removed by the operation of *Lithotomy*.

CALCULI, URETHRAL.—When lodged in the urethra, they obstruct the passage of urine, and occasion a hard tumor, and can be readily recognized by the sound. The only remedy is incision.

CALIGO.—A mist. A speck on the cornea of the eye; Web-eye, Opaque Cornea. It may often be removed by a good surgeon oculist; no one else should meddle with it.

CALLOUS.—Hard or indurated. Ulcers often have callous edges which must be removed with the knife or caustic before they can heal. This is particularly the case with fistulous ulcers.

CANCER.—Carcinoma.   There are many varieties of cancers and ".cancroid growths," but they all consist essentially of a scirrhous, livid tumor, ultimately terminating in a fetid and ichorous ulcer.   Authors distinguish cancerous tumors into 1, *Encephaloid*, which is of a dead white color, and resembles lobulated cerebral matter; 2, *Scirrhus*, which is extremely firm and dense, and resembles the rind of bacon traversed by cellulo-fibrous septa; 3, *Colloid*, when the mass of the tumor, which is firm and resisting, contains a jelly-like matter.   The first-named variety often attains an enormous size, has been observed in almost every tissue and organ of the body, and frequently co-exists in several.   Its progress, especially after ulceration, is usually very rapid.   The second variety generally grows very slowly, and is rarely to be met with larger than an orange.   The third variety is intermediate in its progress, size, and extension.

All forms of cancers are to be treated on the same general plan, yet each may require some modification of it.   In the early stages, and when the tumors are small, repeated congelations will generally arrest their growth, and in some cases, so destroy their vitality as to occasion their removal by absorption.   The best refrigerant is an admixture of snow or pounded ice with salt (two parts of snow or ice to one of salt) which may be applied once a week, for ten, fifteen or twenty minutes, according to the size of the tumor, and the frozen part gradually thawed, under the application of iced-water.   If well managed, this process produces but little pain.   If the tumor cannot be arrested or greatly diminished in size by this means, in two, three or four months (according to its size) the best plan of removal is by means of caustic.   But this can only be managed by a competent physician or attendant, as the material to be selected, and the strength of the preparation, must be adapted to the sensibility of the patient and the *vital* resistance of the diseased mass; otherwise the pain of the process would be unendurable.   Moreover, the kind and strength of the caustic may have to be varied from time to time according to its effects.   Chloride of Zinc, made into a paste with wheat flour, and Anhydrous Sulphate of Zinc, in powder, are among the best articles to disorganize the tumor. To remove very large tumors I prefer to etherize the patient, and apply the strongest caustics, as the concentrated sulphuric acid made into a paste with saffron flowers. While the disorganized portion is being sloughed-off, the part should be covered with an elm-flour poultice.. The caustic should be repeatedly applied, until all vestiges of the tumor and roots are removed, after which it may be dressed with flour and simple cerate.

Meanwhile the general health should be carefully attended to. And it is better not to commence the local treatment until the system has been thoroughly cleansed of the impurities which constitute the cancerous diathesis. For bathing purposes, the wet-sheet pack, the tepid ablution, or the full hot-and-cold bath may be preferable in different states of the circulation. But the temperature of the surface is a sufficient guide in all cases. The diet must be rigidly simple and abstemious. A little of the "Hunger-Cure" would promote the elimination of morbific matters from the system, more rapidly than excessive bathing.

CANINE LAUGH.—Cynic Spasm. *Risus Sardonicus*, Sardonic Smile. The facial expression during laughter, to which this term is applied, is due to a spasmodic contraction of the *Caninus* muscle.

CANTHARADISMUS.—This term will not be found in the Medical Dictionary, but I apply it to the disease occasioned by the application or administration of Spanish flies, whether in the form of blister-plaster, applied to the skin, or of tincture or powder, taken into the stomach. The symptoms are, heat, or a burning pain in the urinary organs, with strangury, or retention of urine, from spasmodic action of the spincter muscles of the bladder. The prolonged warm bath, with frequent sips of warm water, is the remedy.

CAPSICUMISMUS.—The effect of cayenne pepper applied to the living organism, is inflammation; when moderate, it is called "Stimulation," and when severe, "Irritation." In all cases it is disease. And whether "heat is life," and "life a forced state," or heat and force the manifestations of vital action, it is, with me, a clear deduction from the plainest principles of common sense, to say nothing of science, that the heat, stimulation, irritation or inflammation occasioned by *poisons* of any sort, is in no way conducive to health and longevity.

The remedy for the pepper malady is, sips of cool or cold water, bits of ice, and tepid (not cold) ablutions. When there is much heat or burning in the epigastrium from an excessive dose, the wet girdle should be applied. Indeed, pepper to the mucous membrane is what fire is to the skin, and both require the same remedial plan.

CAQUE SANGUE.—An old French term for "Bloody Flux." See Dysentery.

CARBUNCLE.—See Anthrax.

CARBUNCLED FACE.—See Gutta Rosea.

CARBUNCULAR EXANTHEM.—Anthracia. See Plague.

CARDIALGIA.—Gastralgia, Gastrodynia, Heartburn. A gnawing or burning sensation in the stomach or epigastric region. It is a dyspeptic symptom. Sips of warm water will relieve it. Patients who are subject to this symptom should adopt a plain, dry, and sparing diet. Milk, grease and sugar should be eschewed.

CARDIOMALACIA.—*Mollities Cordis.* Softening of the heart.

CARDITIS.—Inflammation of the heart. This is known by intense pain in the region of the heart, throbbing or palpitation, irregular pulse, short, dry cough, and difficult breathing. The pain is increased by pressing upward against the diaphragm, and by lying on either side. There is an insupportable sense of oppression, and the countenance is haggard and anxious. There is also general fever. It is a very rare disease for obvious reasons, except when induced by the maltreatment of gout and rheumatism. The treatment is the same as for Pneumonia, which see.

CARIES.—Ulceration of Bone. It is analogous to *gangrene* of the soft parts. It may result from external injuries or internal cachexia. Mercurial medicines, and other mineral drugs are among the most frequent causes. It is to be treated on the same plan as inflammation of the soft parts. When there is constant heat and pain in the part affected, cold wet cloths should be constantly applied. When there is little or no heat, the warm fomentations two or three times a day, followed by the covered wet compress, should be employed. When the ulcers are deep, they should be cleansed daily and filled with fine flour. The constitutional treatment is of first importance. Pure air, simple diet, and general bathing, according to the superficial temperature, should never be neglected. The Hydro Electrical baths are especially useful in this affection.

CARNIFICATION.—Transformation into flesh; a term applied to a morbid condition of certain organs, in which the tissue acquires a consistence like that of muscle or flesh. When it occurs in the lungs, they present a texture like that of the liver, and are said to be *hepatized*. The bony structure sometimes becomes transformed to a fleshy consistence, as in *osteosarcoma*. Local inflammation, and a general cachectic state of the system, are the causes; hence the remedies are whatever will remove inflammation and purify the body.

CARNOSITAS.—A fleshy excrescence. Nitrate of Silver, Sulphate of Zinc, Nitric acid, or a white-heated iron may be used to destroy it.

CARNOSITIES OF THE URETHRA.—Carbuncles; small, fleshy, fungous growths in the urethra. They are frequently found at the orifice of the female urethra, in persons who have suffered much from acrid leucorrhœa. A few applications of nitric acid, or lunar caustic, will remove them.

CARPHOLOGIA.—A delirious picking of the bed-clothes. In fevers it denotes great irritation of the brain, and is an unfavorable sign. Cold wet cloths should be applied to the head, and warm applications to the feet.

CARPOLOGIA.—See Subsultus Tandinum.

CARUNCLE.—A fleshy excrescence. See Carnositas.

CARUS.—Profound Sleep. Coma, with complete insensibility, so that the patient cannot be aroused, even for an instant. It is always symptomatic. It requires the same treatment as apoplexy.

CATACAUSIS.—Spontaneous combustion of the human body. Cases seem to be well authenticated in which the human.organism will acquire that hydro-carbonaceous condition, in persons who have been long addicted to the excessive use of liquors, that, on the approach of a flame or lighted taper to the mouth, the breath will inflame, and the whole body burn to ashes. It is fire which water will not quench.

CATALEPSY.—A disease characterized by a sudden suspension of the functions of the external senses and of volition, the limbs and trunk preserving the different positions given to them. The fit comes on suddenly, and often ends with singing or whistling. It depends on nervous debility, constipation of the bowels, or congestion of the brain, or all together, and the treatment must have reference to these circumstances.

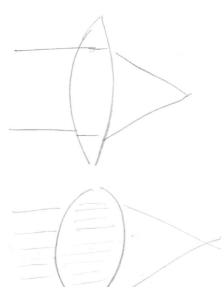

CATARACT.—An opacity of the crystalline lens, or its capsule, which precludes vision. There are many varieties of this affection, for which, the reader who is interested, may consult M. DESMARRES, or any of the standard works on Surgery. The chief causes are, excessive use, or rather abuse, of the eyes, especially by candle or gas-light, and a thick, viscid, bilious state of the blood, the result of unphysiological habits. The disease appears insidiously. At first objects seem misty and indistinct; light bodies float before the eyes, and vision is gradually yet constantly diminished, till finally lost.

If properly treated in the incipient stage, the disease can generally be arrested. The head must be kept cool; the eyes only moderately employed, and not at all after dark; all exciting brain labor must be avoided ; derivative baths—hip

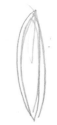

and foot—should be taken daily, and the general bathing and regimen be so adapted to the patient as to purify the mass of blood as rapidly as possible.

CATARRH.—Defluxion, Coryza, Rheuma, Cold, Phlegmatorrhagia. An inflammation of the mucous membrane of the nose and upper portion of the air passages. When caused by exposure, it is called a *common cold*, or *Acute Catarrh*; and when the consequence of a morbid state of the liver, or of constitutional disease or impurity, it is termed *Chronic Catarrh*.

Acute Catarrh can be readily removed by a full warm-bath, followed by a wet-sheet pack, and often by either alone. Warm sitz and foot-baths are proper derivative measures. The patient should fast for a day or two, and remain in an equable temperature.

Chronic Catarrh is almost invariably one of the complications of dyspepsia or liver complaint, and the treatment should be mainly directed to the primary malady. Nasal baths are always more or less useful. A moderate vapor-bath, not so prolonged as to occasion much relaxation, nor any appreciable disturbance of the head, may be employed once or twice a week with especial advantage. In no disease is pure air more indispensable.

CATARRH, EPIDEMIC.—Influenza, which see.

CATARRH, OF THE BLADDER.—An inflammation of the mucous membrane of the bladder, attended with more or less of the fibrinous excretion which takes place in croup and diptheria. The membraneous formation is often expelled in fragments, attended with great pain and difficult micturition. It is to be treated precisely as *Cystitis*, which see.

CATARRH, OF THE BOWELS.—See Diarrhœa Tubular.

CATARRH, OF THE UTERUS.—Membraneous inflammation of the lining membrane of the Uterus, which attends certain forms of mismenstruation. See Dysmenorrhœa.

CATHARSIS.—The purgation of the bowels; usually applied to discharges from the bowels when induced by cathartic medicines. The real disease is diarrhœa, when caused by the "*modus operandi*" of medicinal drugs, or by poisons accidentally introduced, or by impurities casually accumulated. Warm hip-baths, fomentations, frequent sips of cool water, and a quiet, horizontal position, are the remedies.

CAT'S-EYE.—An amaurotic condition. See Amaurosis.

CAULIFLOWER EXCRESCENCE.—An excrescence which appears in the vulva and anus, at or near the origin of the mucous membranes, and which, in appearance, resembles the head of the cauliflower. It is frequently, though not always, of venereal origin. They may be cured by proper cauterization with aquafortis, nitrate of silver, or caustic potassa

CAUMA.—Inflammatory Fever, Synocha.

CAUMATODES.—This and the preceding term have been applied by some authors to Inflammatory or Synochal Fever, which see.

CAUSUS.—A highly ardent fever. PINEL regards it as a complication of bilious and inflammatory fever. BROUSSAIS considers it "an intense-gastritis, accompanied with bilious symptoms." It is properly Synocha, or inflammatory fever.

CAUSUS, INDEMIAL.—Tropicus Endemicus, Yellow Fever of the West Indies. See Yellow Fever.

CENOSIS.—Emaciation, Inanition.

CEPHALÆA.—Periodical Headache, Sick Headache. A nervous headache is caused by acid bile or acidity of the stomach. It may be relieved by drinking plentifully of warm water, and applying the wet-girdle. It is symptomatic of dyspepsia or liver complaint, and can only be permanently relieved by curing the primary malady.

CEPHALÆMATOMA.—Thrombus Neonatorum. A sanguineous tumor which frequently appears on the head of new-born children. It is of little consequence, and usually disappears in a few days.

CEPHALÆNIA.—Cerebral Hyperæmia, Congestion of the head. An accumulation or disproportionate amount of blood in

4

the vessels of the brain, inducing headache, flushed face, with more or less feverishness. Apply cold applications to the head and warm to the feet. If the bowels are constipated, relieve them with enemas of tepid water.

CEPHALAGRA.—Cephalæ Arthritica, Meningitis Arthritica. Gout in the Head. Treat it as recommended in the preceding case.

CEPHALALGIA.—Cephalonia, Encephalgia, Dolor capitis. This term includes every kind of Headache. They are ordinarily symptomatic, and must be relieved by attending to the primary affection. When idiopathic, the treatment advised for the preceding cases are proper.

CEPHALITIS.—Encephalitis, Phænitis, Brain Fever, Inflammation of the Brain. The symptoms are, intense pain in the head, violent fever, redness of the face and eyes, intolerance of light and sound, and delirium.

Apply the coldest water, or what is better, pounded ice, to the head, sponge the surface with tepid or cool water frequently; the bowels, unless already loose, should be freely moved with enemas of tepid water; the head must be well raised on the pillows, and all sources of irritation avoided.

Some authors have applied the term *Meningitis* to inflammation of the membranes of the brain, and *Cerebritis* to inflammation of the substance of the brain. But such distinctions are neither practicable nor useful; and were they so, it would not in the least affect the required treatment.

CEREBELLITIS.—Inflammation of the Cerebellum. This cannot be, and need not be, distinguished from Cephalitis.

CEREBRO-SPINAL MENINGITIS.—This phrase has been applied to a form of putrid typhus, now prevailing in various parts of this country, and often called "spotted fever," on the absurd notion that the disease consists essentially in an inflammation of the coats of the brain and spinal marrow. The ordinary drug treatment is as murderous as the theory is foolish.

CHAFING.—See Intertrigo.

CHLAZA.—A round, hard, transparent tumor developed in the eye-lids and other parts of the body. It requires cauterization. This term is also applied to the *cicatricula* of the egg.

CHANCRE.—Ulcerous Cancrosum. An ulcer resulting from venereal infection, and located on a part of the genital organs. It may be of a phagedenic or rapidly-spreading character, or take the form of deepening ulcers which are filled with an acrid, corroding, and infectious matter. They should be thoroughly cauterized, on their first appearance, with nitric acid or the solid nitrate of silver, and the process repeated as often as there is any appearance of erosive action. Meanwhile, the system should be purified of the syphilitic taint as rapidly as possible by a thorough bathing, and a strict regimen closely bordering on starvation.

CHANCRE LARVE.—A concealed Chancre. RICORD's vagary that such a chancre sometimes exists, and produces virulent gonorrhœa, is, in my opinion, just a vagary and nothing else.

CHRUMOSIS.—*Opthalmia Membranarum.* A form of inflammation of the eye, in which the conjunctiva surrounding the cornea swells so as to form a high ring, causing the cornea to be seen, as it were, at the bottom of a well. For treatment, see Opthalmia.

CHICKEN-POX.—See Varicella.

CHIGGRE.—See Chique.

CHILBLAIN.—Pernio. An erythematous inflammation of the feet, hands, and other parts, caused by extreme and sudden alterations of temperature. Sometimes it degenerates into painful, indolent ulcerations, termed *Kibes*. Keep the part affected in a moderate and equable temperature, and bathe them frequently in tepid or moderately cold water.

CHILD-BED FEVER.—See Puerperal Fever.

CHILD-CROWING.—*Asthma Thymicum.* See Asthma

CHINWHELK.—See Sycosis.

CHIQUE.—Tick, Chiggre, Jigger. A small insect in America and the Antilles, which gets under the scarf skin and produces great irritation.

CHLOASMA. — *Pityriasis Versicoler.* A cutaneous affection characterized by one or more broad, irregular-shaped patches, of a yellow or yellowish-brown color. It occurs most frequently on the front of the neck, breast, abdomen, and groins. It is properly of bilious origin, and may be removed by restoring the action of the liver. The parts affected may be frequently bathed with tepid water, and moderate friction applied afterwards. In this, and in all similar affections of the skin, milk, butter and sugar, should be excluded from the dietary.

CHLOROSIS.—Green Sickness, *Cacheria Virginum.* A morbid condition of young females, particularly those who never menstruated, characterized by pale, lurid complexion, and general debility. Usually there is a capricious and depraved appetite, with constipation of the bowels, and palpitation of the heart. The blood of chlorotic patients is generally deficient in red corpuscles, and physicians dose them with the preparations of iron and other kinds of " blood-food," on the false and absurd notion that these inorganic poisons can supply the deficient elements or in some mysterious way cause them to be manufactured or created.

The patient should exercise as much as possible in the open air. Moderate dancing or the light gymnastics are admirable. The diet should be restricted to coarse bread, ripe fruits, and unseasoned vegetables. A warm bath should be taken once a week; the tepid ablution each other morning on rising; the dry rubbing-sheet on the alternate mornings; the hip-bath of a moderate temperature—90° to 80°—should be taken daily; the hot-and-cold foot-bath at bed-time, and the wet-girdle worn a part of each day when the weather is so warm that it does not occasion chilliness. When there are pains in the loins and back at the time for the menstrual period, the warm hip-bath, or hot fomentations, should be employed until relieved.

CHOLÆMIA.—A bilious condition of blood. See Jaundice.

CHOLCYSTITIS.—Inflammation of the gall-bladder. It cannot be, and need not be, distinguished from Hepatitis, which see.

CHOLELITHUS.—Biliary Calculi. See Calculi.

CHOLER.—Bile, Anger. A superabundance of bile has been supposed to be a cause of the unamiable malady called anger. Take sips of warm water, and repeat the Lord's Prayer.

CHOLERA.—There are several varieties of this disease, all of which are characterized by vomiting and purging, and usually more or less griping in the bowels, with spasms in the legs and arms. The general plan of treatment applicable to all forms is, in the early stages, the tepid rubbing or tepid half-bath, warm hip-baths, hot foot-baths, an enema of warm water to free the bowels, frequent sips of warm water, the wet girdle to the abdomen, and a quiet horizontal posture. In the later stage, the extremities should be kept warm, hot fomentations applied to the abdomen, and hot bottles to the armpits and sides, enemas of a small quantity of cool or cold water should be given once in two or three hours; and when there is a sense of heat or burning about the region of the stomach, small bits of ice may be swallowed occasionally, or sips of iced-water taken. Should there be much heat over the whole surface in the early stage, the tepid or cool wet-sheet pack should be taken, while bottles of hot water are kept to the feet; and if the surface inclines to paleness, and the system to chilliness, the full warm-bath, or vapor-bath, should be given; or, if either is impracticable, hot bottles should be applied to the feet and sides, and fomentations to the abdomen.

CHOLERA, ASIATIC.—See Cholera, Spasmodic.

CHOLERA, ASPHYXIA.—See Cholera, Spasmodic.

CHOLERA, BILIOUS.—Cholera Morbus. So termed, because it is attended with a copious excretion of acrid bile. In the severest cases the vomiting, spasms, and pain, are intense and agonizing, and death often results in a·few hours.

This form of. cholera, though of terrible violence in its symptoms, is scarcely dangerous under proper Hygienic management. At first the patient should drink copiously of warm water, and when the violent retching subsides, take frequent sips of cold water. Cool wet cloths should be applied over the abdomen, extending well up on the chest so as to cover the region of the liver; and if the skin inclines to preternatural heat or feverishness, the whole surface should be sponged with tepid or moderately cold water.

CHOLERA, EPIDEMIC.—See Cholera, Spasmodic.

CHOLERA, EUROPEAN.—See Cholera, Spasmodic.

CHOLERA, FLATULENT.—Wind Cholera, Cholera Sicca. This form is not so dangerous as distressing, and is, characterized by an oppressive flatulence and retching, and an absence of bile in the discharges. · Dyspeptics are very liable to it. Warm water drinking, and fomentations to the abdomen, are the specialities of treatment.

CHOLERA, INDIAN.—See Cholera, Spasmodic.

CHOLERA, INFANTUM.—Infantile Fever, Choleric Fever of Infants, Watery Gripes. This form prevails among children during the warm season. Usually a diarrhœa precedes the vomiting for several days. There is irregular febrile heat, and the body rapidly emaciates.

The full warm-bath should be given at first, after which the wet-girdle (well covered with dry flannel, except when the surface is quite warm and feverish) should be applied to the abdomen; a teaspoonful of cool, but not very cold water, should be given frequently; if the thirst is excessive, tepid water may be allowed with sufficient freedom to allay it; the feet should be kept warm, and the head cool, and the whole surface sponged twice a day with tepid water. An abundance of fresh air must be admitted to the apartment; and if the milk which the child uses is not known to be pure, it should be stopped at once.

CHOLERA, MALIGNANT.—See Cholera, Spasmodic.

CHOLERA, PESTILENTIAL.—See Cholera, Spasmodic.

CHOLERA, SICCA.—See Cholera, Flatulent.

CHOLERA, SPASMODIC.—The Cholera, Rice Disease, the Blue Disease, Cholera Asphyxia, Cholera Typhus, Malignant, Epidemic, Asiatic, Pestilential, European, etc., Cholera. This form of Cholera is characterized by watery discharges from the bowels, blue appearance of the countenance or surface, thirst, spasms in the abdomen and extremities, and, in the later stages, by coldness of the tongue and pulselessness at the wrist.

The treatment must be varied to meet the indications as they present themselves, and the different stages of the malady, and different conditions of the patients. For the early stage, the directions given under the head of Cholera are sufficient. In the stage of prostration or collapse, hot bottles to the feet and sides, or the full hot-bath, followed by the tepid ablution and gentle but active friction, or the warm sitz and hot foot-baths, should be resorted to. The vapor-bath, if practicable, is excellent. The patient should (except when bathing) remain as quietly in bed as possible, and endeavor to restrain rather than promote the ejections. Free ventilation is important. When there is great thirst, frequent draughts of tepid water may be taken, though the quantity taken at a time should be very small. When there is a burning heat in the stomach, bits of ice or sips of iced-water may be frequently taken ; and when the spasms are violent, fomentations should be assiduously applied to the abdomen until relief is obtained. In cases where the warm-bath or vapor-bath is indicated, and impracticable, the warm wet-sheet pack will answer.

CHOLERIC FEVER OF INFANTS —See Cholera Infantum.

CHOLERINE.—The first stage or precursory symptoms of Spasmodic Cholera. The term is usually applied to the premonitory "diarrhoea."

CHOLEROMANIA.—A morbid dread of the Cholera. The charms, amulets, incantations, etc., as assafœtida, mustard, onions, hartshorn, camphor, brandy, salted codfish, dried beef. old cheese, etc., which are employed, even in these enlightened days, and even under the advice of " family physicians," and " Boards of Health," would be ridiculous were they not tragical. They are each and all among the causes of the real cholera.

CHOLEROPHOBIA.—Choleromania, which see.

CHOLERO-TYPHUS.—Spasmodic Cholera.

CHOLESTEATOMA.—A kind of encysted fatty tumor.

CHOLOLITHUS.—See Calculi, Biliary.

CHOLORRHŒA.—An abnormal discharge of bile. The affection is symptomatic of biliousness, sick-headache, cholera morbus, etc.

CHOLOSIS AMERICANA.—Yellow Fever. See Fever, Yellow.

CHOLOZEMIA FEBRILIS.—Bilious Fever. See Fever, Bilious.

CHONDRITIS.—Inflammation of Cartilage.

CHONDROMA.—A morbid growth of cartilage proceeding from bones. Of this nature are, Osteo Sarcoma, spina ventosa, and some other diseases.

CHORDAPSUS.—Intussusception. See Colica-Ileus.

CHORDEE.—A painful inflammation of the urethra attending gonorrhœa. Cold applications are required.

CHOREA.—St. Vitus' Dance, Convulsio Habitualis, Epilepsia Saltatoria, Danse de St. Witt, Danse de St. Guy, Ballismus. A syn-clonic, spasmodic affection, characterized by irregular and involuntary motions of one or more limbs, and of the face and trunk. It is caused by obstruction and debility, and is nearly always preceded by obstinate and prolonged constipation; the use of strong narcotics or nervines, powerful drug medicines, or exhaustive discharges.

In the remedial plan, the dietary is of the first importance. It must be rigidly plain, and very abstemious. Coarse bread and good fruit are the essentials; and the fruit should be largely proportioned to the bread. Passive exercises in the open air are excellent. Abdominal manipulations—kneading, rubbing, etc.—are very useful. The tepid ablution or tepid half-bath should be taken once a day. Moderate douching along the spine may be advantageous. All disturbing mental influences should be specially guarded against. The Sitz-bath at 80° to 85° should be employed for ten minutes once or twice a day, by those who are not deficient in external temperature.

CHRONIC DISEASE.—The term, chronic, applied to disease, means, of long duration. But in a stricter sense it applies to any disease which does not tend to terminate in a limited time by a crisis, at which the patient manifestly begins to sink, or becomes convalescent. Thus, Dyspepsia, Consumption, Diabetis, Jaundice, Neuralgia, etc., are *chronic* diseases; while fevers, and visceral inflammations of all kinds, are its antithesis—*acute.*

CHTHONOPHAGIA.—The negroes of the South, and of the West Indies, are sometimes affected with a morbid craving, and an irresistible propensity to eat earth. It is a malady of the nutritive functions. For the treatment, see Chlorosis.

CHYLURIA.—A discharge of milky urine, without apparent structural disease of the bladder or kidneys. See Diabetis.

CICATRIZATION.—The process by which a scar is formed on wounded or ulcerated surfaces. Every tissue, except the cuticle, hair, nails, and enamel, is supposed to be capable of cicatrization. A scar or cicatrix may vary much in consistence, shape and thickness. The cicatrix of bone is called *Callus.* The scars, after small-pox, are called *pits* or *pock-marks.* To prevent unseemly pitting and scarring after eruptive fevers, burns, scalds, etc., the ulcerated surface should be protected from the contact of the atmosphere. Fine flour is one of the best appliances for this purpose.

CINCHONISM.—The disease resulting from the medicinal use of Peruvian Bark. See Quininism.   4*

CIRCUMGYRATIO.—See Vertigo.

CIRRHOSIS.—A term applied to a morbid condition in which a yellow coloring matter is formed in the tissues. It is undoubtedly owing to deficient action of the liver, in connection with a plethoric or cachectic state of the whole system. A tepid ablution daily, a spare and simple dietary, the hip-bath once or twice a day, and the wet-girdle, are the remedies.

CIRSOCELE.—Cirsocele, Varicose Hernia. The varicose dilatation of the spermatic veins. The scrotum feels as if it contained earth-worms. Many authors confound this affection with *Varicocele*, which is a tumor formed by the veins of the scrotum. These complaints can generally be cured in the early stages, by a strict diet, cold hip-baths, the fountain-bath, cold compresses, etc. It is always advisable to wear the suspensory bandage.

CIRSOMPHALUS.—Varicose dilatation of the veins surrounding the navel.

CLAVUS.— This term is variously applied to warts, corns, condylomatous excrescences of the uterus, and callous tumors of the white of the eye.

CLAVUS HYSTERICUS.— An acute pain in the head, compared by the patients to a sensation as if a nail were driven into the head. It is always symptomatic, and may be relieved by attending to the primary affection. See Headache.

CLIMATIC DISEASES.— The climate is accused of causing many diseases, which are due solely to the habits of the people. Indeed, if people in all climates would live as hygienic as possible, we should hear very little of climatic diseases.

CLONIC.—A term applied to convulsive motions, attended with alternate contraction, and relaxation, in contradistinction to *Tonic* Spasm, when the contractions are continuous and the parts rigid. Epilepsy, palpitation, winking, yawning, etc., are examples.

CNIDOSIS.—A pungent itching. See Urticaria.

COPOCELE, CODOSCELLA.—See Bubo.

CŒLIAC FLUX, CŒLIAC PASSION. — Licutery. A species of diarrhœa in which the food is discharged in an undigested condition. It is symptomatic of Dyspepsia, tuberculosis and other affections. See Diarrhœa.

COLD. — The simple feeling of cold in its various degrees is called *chilliness* and shivering. The disease commonly denominated a cold, is the inflammatory or feverish condition consequent on being exposed to sudden and extreme alterations of temperature. It is attended with more or less sense of stiffness in the muscles, and some degree of soreness about the head and mucous membranes of the nose, throat, and windpipe.

The warm-bath, when the body is cold, and the wet-sheet pack, when the body is hot, with hot foot-baths frequently, cool applications to the head, and the "hunger-cure" dietary, are the remedies for colds.

COLIC. — Colicus, Colique, Belly-ache, Gripes. This disease, of which there are several forms, is characterized by griping pains in the abdomen, with vomiting and costiveness. The general plan of treatment consists in moving the bowels freely with enemas of tepid water; the application of fomentations to the abdomen; draughts of warm water taken freely, and such other warm, tepid or cold applications, as the general temperature demands.

COLIC, OF CONSTIPATION. — This is caused by indurated feces, and requires a plain diet, mostly frugivorous, hip-baths, abdominal manipulations, and tepid enemas, perseveringly employed.

COLIC, CONSTRICTIVE. — This results from a stricture in some part of the alimentary canal, occasioned by a thickening of the mucous membrane. It is known by discharges of liquid stools, and occasionally, after a great effort, solid feces of a very slender caliber. A rigidly abstemious dietary, free exercise in the open air, and the careful avoidance of salt, pepper, spices, and all irritating causes, will generally overcome the difficulty in time.

COLIC, CONVULSIVE.—Spasmodic Colic, Iliac Passion, Intus-susception, Stercoraceous Colic. In this form of Colic one portion of the bowel passes into another, and, by becoming swollen and inflamed, becomes, as it were, fastened in the abnormal position. The vomiting is exceedingly violent, ejecting bile from the duodenum, and often fecal matter from the bowels. Constipation is always the predisposing cause, while the act of vomiting, attended with spasmodic contraction, may be the exciting cause of the displacement. Females, in the early stages of pregnancy, who are constipated, and are, from any cause, excited to vomiting, are very liable to intussusception as a complication. There is always in intussusception a hardness and tenderness, readily noticeable on pressure with the hand near the umbilicus.

The patient should take frequent sips of very cold water; cold wet cloths should be applied over the umbilical region; the bowels must be moved, and kept free, by means of enemas of tepid water, and the patient kept as still and quiet as possible.

COLIC, FLATULENT.—Wind Colic. Warm water drinking, and fomentations to the abdomen, are all that this form of the disease requires, except it be an enema.

COLIC, METALLIC.—Lead Cholic, Devonshire Cholic, Plumbers' Colic, Painters' Colic, Rachialgia, Colic Pictonum, Dry Bellyache. This species of Colic is caused by the introduction of lead into the system, either as medicine, or by its absorption while engaged in the avocation of painting. It is known by a pain at the pit of the stomach, at first dull and remittent, but gradually becoming more violent and continued, extending upward to the arms, and downward to the navel, back, loins, etc. The patient often feels as if some one were cutting him through with a knife. The bowels are usually obstinately constipated, and often loaded with hard, fecal lumps, called Scybala.

The hot or vapor-bath, followed by a tepid spray, ablution, or the rubbing-sheet, should be administered daily, or every other day. Fomentations should be applied to the painful parts; the bowels relieved with copious enemas of tepid or warm water. In cases where there is a comparatively good external circulation, the wet-sheet pack will be even more beneficial than the hot or vapor bath. The dietary should be restricted to coarse bread, gruels, ripe fruit, and a moderate allowance of vegetables. The Electro-Chemical, or Hydro-Electrical baths, though not specifics for metallic poisonings, are highly beneficial auxiliaries in the treatment.

COLIC, OF SURFEIT.—Colica Cibaria. This is occasioned by irritating or indigestible aliment, or by over-eating. Shell fish often induce it in the warm season. Old cheese, stale pork, sausages, semi-putrescent poultry, sometimes occasion it. It is characterized by extreme nausea, with dizziness, a sense of constriction in the throat, and an intolerable sense of suffocation.

The stomach should be relieved by warm water drinking until retching subsides. The bowels should be moved with copious enemas, after which rest and cold wet cloths to the epigastrium will be sufficient.

COLITIS.—Inflammation of that portion of the intestinal tube termed the colon. It may be treated as Enteritis, of which it is a part.

COLLIQUATIVE.—A term applied to various discharges which seem rapidly to exhaust the system, as *Colliquative Diarrhœa* in the later stages of consumption; *Colliquative Sweats* in low fevers, etc.

COLONITIS.—Dysentery, which see.

COLPORRHŒA.—See Leucorrhœa.

COMA.—Profound Sleep. It is a symptom in many diseases, and indicates extreme congestion of the brain, or the effect of narcotic drugs. In some cases it is attended with delirium. Apply cold applications to the head, and warm to the feet, and keep the patient quiet in a well-ventilated room.

COMBUSTION, SPONTANEOUS, OR HUMAN.—Preternatural Combustibility. See Catacausis.

COMMOTION.—See Concussion of the Brain.

COMPLICATION.—In pathology, this means the co-existence of several maladies, or the supervention of several diseases which are no part of the primary affection. Thus, if a person has a fever and takes large doses of opium, calomel, antimony, and jalap, he will have, in addition to the fever, congestion of the brain, ulceration of the mouth, inflammation of the intestines, and diarrhœa. Nine-tenths of all the complications which so embarrass the physicians and destroy the patients, are really drug diseases.

COMPRESSION OF THE BRAIN.—This may arise from effusion, extravasation, a soft tumor, or wounds and injuries by which a portion of the skull-bone is depressed, or a foreign body lodged upon, or within the brain. The symptoms are of the apoplectic and comatose character. It is to be treated as apoplexy and coma, except where surgical treatment is required.

CONCUSSION OF THE BRAIN.— Stunning, Shock. In severe cases there is a complete loss of sensation and voluntary motion. It is induced by blows, falls, or other sudden injuries, and requires the same treatment as apoplexy, coma, etc.

CONFLUENT.—A term applied to small-pox, and measles, in which the pustules and pimples run together. It indicates the low, typhoid, and most dangerous form of those diseases.

CONGENITAL.—Diseases or mal-conformations which exist from birth.

CONGESTION.—Accumulation of Blood, Engorgement, and Disproportionate Dilatation of the Blood-Vessels. A great degree of congestion is called *Stagnation*. In all diseases the circulation of the blood is more or less unbalanced, hence there must of necessity be a greater or less degree of congestion. In high or entonic fevers, the superficial capillary vessels are in a state of congestion; and in all low or atonic fevers, and in all chronic diseases, some one or more of the internal organs are congested. In inflammatory diseases, the organ or part inflamed is the seat of congestion. Hence congestion is always symptomatic, and the treatment must have reference to the primary disease. The principle applicable to the treatment of all forms of congestion is, to induce determination of the blood *from* the part affected. Thus, when the head or lungs are congested, warm hip-baths, the wet-girdle, and hot foot-baths, are proper derivatives, or, in medical parlance, "counter-irritants."

CONGESTIVE FEVER.—This term has been applied to various forms of low fever, of the intermittent, remittent, and continued type, in which there is engorgement and disproportionate functional disturbance of the brain or lungs.

CONJUNCTURITIS.—Inflammation of the mucous membrane which covers the interior surface of the eye. It is sometimes termed *Catarrhal*, *Purulent*, and *Egyptian* Opthalmia. See Opthalmia.

CONSENSIS.—Consent of parts, Sympathy. A vagary of the imaginations of medical men, which has no other existence in nature.

CONSTIPATION.—Costiveness, Alvine Obstruction, Fecal Retention. This is the most prevalent morbid condition of the people of the civilized world; and it is the parent-source of more disease, impurity, dissipation, premature death, and human misery, than all other maladies that can be named. And so long as the present eating habits of the people continue, constipation, and all its train of putrid fevers, choleras, dyspepsias, convulsions, consumptions, nervous debilities, anæmias, etc., must fill the land with invalids and people the graveyards with victims. There is no remedy for constipation, except in the adoption of a plain, simple, unstimulating diet, and a due amount of exercise. In order to overcome confirmed habits of constipation, the diet should be largely frugivorous, enemas should be employed when necessary, hip-baths should be employed frequently, and such exercises as call into activity the abdominal and respiratory muscles, should be perseveringly resorted to. The "Swedish movements" are excellent.

CONSUMPTION.—Phthisis, Phthisis-Pulmonalis. In a strict and proper sense, this term is applied to all forms of chronic inflammation of the pulmonary apparatus, attended with structural disorganization. The disease is known by cough, difficulty or shortness of breathing, expectoration, pain or sense of weight in the chest, and, in the later stages, emacia-tion, and hectic fever. There are no less than seven distinct forms of consumption, notwithstanding most authors recognize but two or three, and some but a single form—the Tubercular. The essential nature of consumption is an effort of the system to relieve the blood-vessels of effete matter, poisons, or impu-rities through the lungs, inducing obstruction, inflammation, hemorrhage, tuberculation, etc. Whatever tends to lower the tone of the vital powers, and diminish the functional activity of the other excretory organs, and especially whatever tends to weaken the respiratory function, as foul air, sedentary habits, overloaded stomachs, stimulating viands, etc., are among the producing causes of this prevalent and increasing malady.

In the general remedial plan, pure air, with regular and persistent exercise, are of first importance. Such exercises as tend to develop the muscles of the chest and expand the lungs, should be especially attended to, as rowing, pulling, rotating the arms with the light dumb-bells, etc. Horseback riding is excellent in the early stages. The patient should keep the body in as equable a temperature as possible, and carefully avoid overheated rooms. The dietary can hardly be too sim-ple; and when the lungs are much ulcerated or tuberculated, it should be rather abstemious. Milk, butter, cheese, sugar, fat, alcohol, lard, pork, cod-liver oil, and all such abominations of "Hydro-carbons," although now recommended by a ma-jority of physicians as remedial, should be carefully abstained from. Consumptives should never take more than two meals per day. The bathing appliances should be governed by the particular circumstances of each case, and will be noticed in the following varieties.

CONSUMPTION, APOSTEMATOSIS.—This consists of an abscess—aposteme—formed in the substance or parenchyma of the lungs. It is attended with a fixed pain, dry cough, and diffi-culty of lying on one side. The cough at length terminates in a sudden and copious expectoration. The abscess may then heal, to be followed sooner or later by another.

This form of consumption is perhaps the least dangerous, and most readily curable of all. The patient should wear the chest-wrapper, whenever he can do so without permanent chilliness; take a tepid ablution, half-bath, or the wet-sheet pack, daily, and a hip-bath at 80° to 85°, ten minutes, towards evening, with a hot-and-cold foot-bath at bedtime.

CONSUMPTION, BRONCHIAL.—This is the Chronic Bronchitis of authors. Acute Bronchitis is but another name for Pneumonia. Bronchial consumption consists in a chronic inflammation of the mucous membrane of the bronchial ramifications, and is characterized by a diffused sense of heat and soreness in the chest, increased on a full inspiration, moderate cough, with more or less expectoration. It is easily cured in the early stages, and should be treated precisely as recommended for the apostematous variety. In the later stages, when the patient is much reduced, the dry rubbing-sheet, in the morning, the tepid half-bath—85° to 90°—for five minutes, at noon, the hip-bath—85° to 80°—for ten minutes, at four to five, P. M., and the hot-and-cold foot-bath, for ten minutes, at bedtime, will be adapted to the majority of cases.

CONSUMPTION, CATARRHAL.—In this form the cough is frequent and violent, and the expectoration copious. The cough is also deep and resonant. It is the sequel of repeated colds and catarrhal affections. It is quite curable in the early stage, and often in seemingly desperate cases. The plan of treatment is precisely the same as recommended for the preceding two varieties.

CONSUMPTION, DYSPEPTIC.—This variety is so named, because it supervenes upon a prior dyspeptic condition. It is always preceded by a diseased liver. This is the most prevalent form of consumption.

In its treatment, the digestive organs, the liver particularly, must be especially regarded. The diet should be nearly limited to good fruit and unleavened bread. Fomentations should be applied over the region of the liver for ten minutes daily, or semi-weekly. Hip and foot-baths, of a moderate temperature, should be employed daily. The wet-sheet pack, or tepid ablution may be employed daily, or each other day, according to the superficial temperature, and which is preferable, should be determined by the heat of the body. "Swedish movements" applied to the abdominal and respiratory muscles are of great benefit. When the patient is disposed in the forepart of the day, the dry rubbing-sheet is the proper morning application.

CONSUMPTION, HEMORRHAGIC.—This is sometimes called the "galloping consumption." It is characterized by repeated attacks of pæmoptysis, or spitting of blood. It indicates extreme laxity of tissue, and is one of the most difficult varieties to cure.

The patient must remain much in the open air, but be careful to preserve an equable and agreeable temperature of body by means of proper clothing. The exercises should be very gentle, and mostly passive, as sailing, carriage-riding, etc. The diet must be very simple and quite abstemious. Whenever hemorrhage occurs, the patient should remain quiet, in a moderately recumbent posture, and take frequent sips of cold or iced-water until the bleeding ceases. The extremities must at all times be kept warm. Hip and foot-baths are important derivatives. When there is much sensation of heat in the chest, a wet towel, covered with dry flannel, should be laid over it, and frequently changed.

CONSUMPTION, LARYNGEAL.—This is usually among the segnetæ or complications of some of the other forms of the disease, in their later stages; but it sometimes occurs as the primary affection. It is characterized by soreness at the upper part of the windpipe; hoarseness, which is usually quite variable; sense of tickling or irritation, which is sometimes excessive; and muco-purulent expectoration, which is often streaked with blood.

It is to be treated precisely as the dyspeptic form, with the exception that the throat should be frequently bathed with cold water, followed by active friction with dry flannel; and, whenever there is much heat or soreness in the larynx, wet cloths, covered with dry, should be applied around the throat during the night. When the cough is very troublesome, frequent sips of warm water will relieve it.

CONSUMPTION, TUBERCULAR.—This is the only form of consumption recognized by some authors. Next to the dyspeptic form it is the most prevalent. Indeed, in a majority of cases of dyspeptic consumption, the lungs become more or less tuberculated as the disease progresses. It is characterized by a short, tickling cough, sense of weight, fullness, heaviness, or stricture in the upper part of the chest; the breathing is short, and a full inspiration difficult, if not impossible; expectoration scanty and adhesive, except in the later stages. Curdy, cheesy, or earthy particles are often found in the sputa. Tubercular Consumption is usually, though not always, connected with the scrofulous diathesis. It may be regarded as the most intractable form of the disease.

In the treatment, every measure and expedient which can expand the lungs and increase "the breath of life," should be resorted to. How much the patient can exercise with benefit, as well as what exercises will be the most advantageous, will depend on the degree of obstruction in the lungs. Exercises should never be of a kind nor so violent as to occasion panting or palpitation, nor seriously disturb the respiration and circulation. Derivative hip and foot-baths are always indicated; but the kind and temperature of the general baths must, as mentioned in the preceding varieties, be selected according to the temperature or feverishness of the patient.

NOTE.—It should be remarked that two or more forms of consumption often co-exist, and there is a tendency in all forms to become more or less complicated with tubercular deposits and laryngeal inflammation, in the progress of the disease. Laryngitis supervening on any other form, is always a very unfavorable symptom.

CONTAGIOUS DISEASES.—Diseases whose *causes* are capable of being communicated through the atmosphere, or by contact, as small-pox, measles, whooping-cough, mumps, etc. If slaughterhouses, stables, pig-stys, henneries, etc., and the use of animal food, were abolished, contagious diseases would soon disappear.

CONTINUED FEVER.—A fever whose paroxyms have neither remissions nor intermissions until it reaches the crisis. Typhoid, inflammatory, and eruptive fevers, are of the continued type.

CONTRACTURA.—Ectasia, Muscular Stiff-Joint, Permanent rigidity of the flexor muscles which prevents or limits the action of the extensor muscles. The affected muscles form hard cords beneath the skin. It is a frequent sequel of rheumatic affections, and mercurial or other mineral medicines are its most common causes. Hot fomentations, attended with the cool or cold douche, the vapor-bath, and friction, are the remedial measures. The Hydro-Electrical bath is applicable specially to these cases.

CONTUSION.—An injury occasioned by a blunt instrument. When slight and accompanied with an extravasation of blood, it is called a *bruise;* when the skin is divided or broken, the injury is termed a *contused wound.* Cold applications are generally sufficient. When the circulation is low, warm fomentations, followed by cold wet cloths, are advisable.

CONVERSION OF DISEASES. —By this phrase, the Medical Lexicons mean "the change or transformation of one disease into another." This notion is based on the popular and professional fallacy that disease is a substance, or entity.

CONVULSIO CEREALIS.—Raphania, Ergotismus Spasmodicus. A spasmodic affection attended with a peculiar tingling and formication in the arms and legs. It has prevailed endemically in some parts of Germany, and has been attributed to the use of damaged or diseased grain.

CONVULSIONS.—Eclampsia, Spasms, Fits, Cramp, Irregular Muscular Contractions. The class of convulsive diseases is very extensive, embracing no less than five distinct groups of spasmodic affections, termed respectively, the *Comatose,* the

Synclonic, the *Suffocative*, the *Clonic*, and the *Constrictive* or *Tonic Spasm*. Examples of each are, *Epilepsy*, St. *Vitus' Dance*, *Asthma*, *Hiccough*, and *Lock-Jaw*. The diseases of the different groups will be treated of under their respective popular names.

CONVULSION, INFANTILE.—These are almost invariably the effect of indigestible food or constipated bowels; and as, under prevailing fashion, the children are fed worse and worse, deaths of convulsions are becoming more and more frequent. An enema of tepid water to free the bowels, a warm-bath, followed by perfect quiet, constitute the remedial plan.

CONVULSIONNAIRE. — A French word which was applied, during the last century, to persons who had, or pretended to have, convulsions induced by religious impulses. See Dancing Mania.

CONVULSIONS, PUERPERAL.—So denominated when the convulsions affect women in a state of pregnancy, during labor, or in child-bed. They may be occasioned by plethora, constipation, local irritations, mental shocks, etc.

The bowels should be freely moved, cold applications made to the head, warm to the feet, and, unless contra-indicated by inflammation or hemorrhage, fomentations to the abdomen.

COPHOSIS, COPHOTES.—Deafness.

COPPER-NOSE.—Gutta Rosea, which see.

COPROPHORESIS, COPRORRHŒA.—Diarrhœa, Catharsis.

COPROSTASIS.—Constipation.

CORDEE.—Chordee.

CORN.—Clavus. A small, hard tumor which forms on the foot, and commonly on the toes. It is almost always induced by the pressure of tight shoes or boots. They may be destroyed by soaking the part in warm water occasionally, and afterward touching the tumor with caustic, or nitric acid, nitrate of silver, or sulphate of zinc.

CORPULENCE.—Obesity, Polysarcia, Fleshy. An excess of adipose matter, resulting from excessive or abnormal alimentation, with retention of effete or waste matters. The remedy is spare diet, with active exercise.

CORROSION.—DUNGLISON's Medical Dictionary defines this word, "The *action* or *effect* of corrosive substances." When medical men learn to distinguish between *actions, effects,* and *causes,* we shall have a new and perhaps a true medical science. Those who wish to read a discussion involving this subject, are referred to my recent work, "The True Temperance Platform." My forthcoming work, "Principles of Hygienic Medication," will contain a more complete exposition of the problems concerned.

CORRUPTION.—This word is sometimes applied to the purulent matter of a boil, abscess, or ulcer, and sometimes to organic matter in a state of putrefactive decomposition. DUNGLISON defines the term, "Reaction of the particles of a body on each other;" and says, "it is probable that something like corruption may take place even in the living body." A recognition of the true distinction between vital actions and chemical changes, shows at once the *impossibility* of anything like corruption in a living body. Living things never putrefy until after they die.

CORYZA.—Nasal Catarrh, Cold in the Head. Inflammation, with a mucus, or muco-purulent, discharge from the lining membrane of the nasal cavities, and the sinuses communicating therewith.

Rest, abstinence, an equable temperature, and warm footbaths, are the remedies. When the whole system is feverish, a full warm-bath, or wet-sheet pack, is advisable.

COUGH.—Tussis. A spasmodic and sonorous expiratory action of the respiratory apparatus. It is symptomatic of many diseases, and but rarely idiopathic. To suppress it with opiates, as is too much the fashion in asthmatic consumption, etc., is, to say the least, a very dangerous practice. It should be cured by removing the cause; that is, treating the primary malady.

COUGH, HOOPING.—See Pertussis.

COUGH, WINTER.—A term applied to Chronic Bronchitis.

COUNTER-IRRITATION.—A morbid condition induced by remedial agents in one part or organ of the body, in order to relieve irritation or disease in another part or organ. Vesicants and caustics, of various degrees of potency, as mustard, vinegar, cayenne-pepper, alcohol, nitric acid, nitrate of silver, arsenic, corrosive sublimate, chloride of zinc, salts of potassa and lime, sulphate of zinc, mercurials, etc., etc., are chiefly used for this purpose.

These drug diseases are to be treated precisely as Burns or Scalds, which see.

COUP DE SOLEIL.—Sun-Stroke. Sudden congestion or inflammation of the brain, occasioned by exposure to the direct heat of the sun. The condition and symptoms closely resemble those of apoplexy, and the malady requires the same plan of treatment.

COURAP.—An eruption on the skin, attended with perpetual itching. It is common in India, and is due to a bilious condition of the blood. The remedies are, plain food, and a daily ablution.

COWPOX.—See Vaccina.

COXALGIA.—Coxitis, Coxarthritis. Terms applied to pain in the hip, usually of a rheumatic nature or origin. Fomentation will relieve it.

COXARUM MORBUS.—Hip-Disease. Caries of the head of the thigh bone, (os femoris,) often attended with displacement of the head of the bone and shortening of the limb. Persons of a scrofulous diathesis are most liable to this affection.

The local inflammation is to be treated with cold wet cloths, so long as there is preternatural heat, while all the appliances of Hygiene should be resorted to, in order to renovate the whole system as rapidly as possible. A light room, plenty of sunshine, and an abundance of fresh air, are indispensable. Hard water should not be drunk, nor should milk be allowed.

Even sugar is injurious. · The dietary should be very simple, largely frugivorous, and mostly solid. Broths, gruels, soups, mushes, etc., are specially objectionable. The skin should be invigorated with a daily ablution, and, if practicable, exposed to air and sunshine afterwards.

After the inflammation has subsided, the deformity can frequently be partially, and sometimes completely, remedied by a surgical operation.

CRABLOUSE.—A species of Pediculus, which infests the pudendum and axilla. Anguintum or citron ointment will speedily destroy them.

CRABYAWS.—An ulcer on the soles of the feet, with edges so hard as to be cut with difficulty. It is .peculiar to the West Indies.

CRAMP.—Sudden, spasmodic, and painful contraction of one or more muscles. Friction, compression, and fomentations are the remedies. Cramp is symptomatic of some diseases, as *colica pictornum, cholera morbus*, etc.

CRAMP, OF THE STOMACH.—An extremely painful affection of the stomach, with a sense of constriction in the epigastric region. Acid bile, and other irritants, may cause it. Copious warm-water drinking, hot fomentations, and the warm hip-bath are the remedies.

CRAMP, WRITERS'.—Stammering of the Fingers; an irregular contraction of the fingers, so that they are unable to govern or even hold the pen, pencil, or brush. It is caused by too intense or prolonged use of the fingers, in a particular manner. The exciting cause is not unfrequently, an overloaded stomach. Rest, "temperance in all things," and variety of exercise, are all that we need say of remedial measures.

CRAZINESS.—See Insanity.

CRETINISM.—A state of idiocy, commonly accompanied with an enormous goitre. It is epidemic in the low vallies of Switzerland, Tyrol, and the Pyrenees.

Mentally, the Cretin should be treated as we educate idiots; and bodily, he should be treated as we manage the scrofulous diathesis. These unfortunate creatures rarely attain an advanced age.

CRICK, IN THE NECK.—A painful rheumatic affection of the muscles of the neck, causing the patient to incline the head to one side. Fomentations, and friction, will remedy the difficulty.

CRISIS.—A prominent change, for better or worse, in the symptoms of a disease; or a new manifestation of remedial action. Patients, under Hygienic treatment, often have feverish paroxysms, eruptions of the skin, boils, diarrhœa, etc., which are to be regarded as critical efforts. Some patients have many crises during the process of cure, while others recover perfectly, with nothing of the kind. The rule of practice is, to suspend very active treatment. Give the patient more rest, and treat the symptoms with soothing appliances.

CRITICAL DAYS.—Days on which fevers are most likely to terminate. The ancient physicians could predict, with comparative certainty, the duration of the different forms of fevers; but the modern doctors have so shattered the remedial action, and complicated the original malady, with the superinduced drug diseases, that critical periods are almost wholly disregarded. As a general rule, it may be stated that, when left to themselves, inflammatory fevers and visceral inflammations have an average duration of one week; putrid fevers, two weeks, and nervous fevers, three weeks. Maltreatment or accidental complications, and constant dosing and drugging, may prolong their duration to six, eight, ten or twelve weeks.

CRITICAL PERIOD.—The cessation of the menstrual flux, usually called the "*Turn of Life.*" See Mismenstruation.

CROUP.—*Cynanche trachealis*, Hives, Rising of the Lights, Stuffing. Inflammation of the mucous membrane of the windpipe, attended with an excretion of coagulable lymph, which often concretes into a membraneous structure, and induces death by suffocation. The harsh voice, sonorous and suffocative breathing, and shrill, ringing, or barking cough, afford an unerring diagnosis. Says DUNGLISON, "The fever is always highly inflammatory." This is a grave mistake. The fever which attends croup is invariably of the low or typhoid diathesis.

As the local affection, and also the constitutional, febrile disturbance have all degrees of severity and debility, the treatment must be varied accordingly. It is always proper, and generally indispensable, in the outset, to apply cold wet cloths to the throat, to be frequently changed until the preternatural heat subsides. If this is promptly and thoroughly attended to, the excretion will be arrested, and the formation of the *false membrane* prevented. If there is much heat of the whole surface, the tepid half-bath or wet-sheet-pack should be employed; if not the warm bath should be preferred. After bathing, the patient should be placed in bed, and gentle perspiration encouraged. The feet should be kept warm, and the bowels free. When the cough is tight and suffocative, and expectoration difficult, warm water may be drunk moderately, and fomentations applied to the chest. When there is great thirst, with sense of heat in the mouth, throat, or chest, the patient may be allowed frequent sips of cold or iced water.

CROUP, HYSTERIC.—A spasmodic affection of the laryngeal muscles, which frequently affects hysterical females. It can be relieved by fomentations to the throat and abdomen.

CROUP, PSEUDO.—Dry Asthma. See Asthma.

CRUSTA.—A Crust or Scab. An assemblage of small flakes, formed by the drying up of a fluid, excreted by the skin.

CRUSTA LACTEA.—See Porrigo Larvalis.

CRUSTA GENU EQUINÆ.—Sweat or Knee Scab, Hangers, Dew Claws, Night Eyes, Horse Crust. A morbid secretion of the horse.

CRUSTULA.—A small shell or scab. An ecchymosis of the conjunctiva, is so called.

CURVATURE.—A bending or crooking of any part of the body. The common causes are, relaxation of the muscles and caries of the bones. Spinal curvatures are very prevalent in these days of dyspeptic stomachs, and constipated bowels. The curvature may be forward, backward, or lateral.

In addition to all the ordinary Hygienic appliances, for invigorating the whole muscular system, various gymnastic exercises, and particularly the "Swedish Movements," as modified and improved by the Hygeio-Therapeutic physicians, are of inestimable value.

CUT.—A solution of continuity, made by a sharp instrument. Bring the divided parts together as accurately as possible; retain them there by adhesive plaster or sutures, and keep the morbid heat down with cold compresses.

CUTANEOUS DISEASES.—The various *eruptions of the skin* are naturally grouped into the following genera and species:

1. EXANTHEMATOUS........... { Urticaria, Roseola, Erythema.

2. VESICULAR................... { Pemphigus, Rupia, Herpes, Eczema.

3. PUSTULAR.................... { Impetigo, Ecthyma, Scabies.

4. PAPULAR.................... { Lichen, Strophulus, Prurigo.

5. SQUAMOUS.................. { Lepra, Psoriasis, Pityriasis.

6. FOLLICULOUS.............. { Acne, Sycosis, Ichthyosis, Trichosis, Favus.

They will be treated of under their common or specific names.

CUTITIS, CYTITIS.—Terms applied to erysipelatous inflammation.

CYANOPATHY, CYANOSIS.—Kyanosis, Blue Malady. These terms are applied to a morbid condition in which the surface of the body is colored blue. It commonly depends on a direct communication between the cavities of the right and left sides of the heart, in consequence of which a portion of venous blood is not carried to the lungs for aeration. This communication may exist, however, without occasioning the blueness.

CYNANCHE.—Angina, Isthmitis, Paristhmitis, Sore Throat, Paracynanche, Dog Choak. Inflammation of the throat and upper portion of the air passages.

CYNANCHE, EPIDEMICA.—Mumps. See Parotis.

CYNANCHE, MALIGNA.—Putrid Sore Throat. It is properly malignant scarlet fever. See Scarlatina, Maligna.

CYNANCHE, PAROTIDÆ.—See Parotis.

CYNANCHE, PHARYNGEA.—See Quinsy.

CYNANCHE, TONSILLARIS.—Tonsillitis. See Quinsy.

CYNANCHE, TRACHEALIS.—See Croup.

CYSTALGIA.—Pain in the Bladder. It may be occasioned by retention of urine, gravel, stone, or catarrhal inflammation, venereal infection, or diuretic medicines or beverages, and should be treated accordingly.

CYSTIRRHŒA.—Catarrh of the Bladder. A copious discharge of mucus from the bladder with the urine, attended with Dysuria. It depends on chronic inflammation of the mucous membrane. The excretion is often fibrinous, concreting into a preternatural membrane, which is cut off and expelled in fragments. For the treatment, see Cystitis.

CYSTITIS.—Acute Inflammation of the Bladder. When chronic, it is called Catarrh of the Bladder, and Cystirrhœa. Frequent tepid or cool hip-baths, the wet-girdle, and, when feverish, the wet-sheet pack, or the full warm-bath, are the proper bathing appliances. The diet must be abstemious in the acute form, and very plain and simple in the chronic or catarrhal form.

CYSTOCELE.—Hernia of the Bladder. The tumor is soft and fluctuating; disappears on pressure, and increases in size when the urine is retained. The remedy is a truss.

CYSTODYNIA.—Rheumatic Pain of the Bladder. Fomentations, or warm hip-baths, will relieve it.

CYSTOPARALYSIS.—Paralysis of the Bladder. See Eneuresis.

CYSTORRHAGIA.—A discharge of blood from the vessels of the urinary bladder. See Hæmaturia.

CYTITIS.—Inflammation of the skin.

DACRYOPS.—An obstruction and swelling of the lachrymal passages, inducing what is called "weeping-eye." It is an inflammatory condition, and requires cold applications.

DACRYOSOLENITIS.—Inflammation of the lachrymal ducts.

DANCING MANIA.—Dancing Plague. An epidemic, convulsive affection, which appeared at various times in the Middle Ages, under the names of St. Vitus' Dance, St. John's Dance, Tarantism, Hysteria, Tigretier, etc. It was no doubt extended sympathetically. "Moral and legal suasion," in the form of "coercion," were found the most effectual remedies. For a complete history of the strange malady, the reader is referred to HECKER's "Epidemics of the Middle Ages."

DANDRIFF, DANDRUFF.—See Pityriasis.

DANDY.—See Dengue.

DARTRE.—See Herped.

DAYMARE.—See Incubus.

DAY-SIGHT.—See Hemoralopia.

DEAF-DUMBNESS.—Mutitas Surdorum, Aphonia Surdorum. Speechlessness from deafness. It may be congenital or accidental.

DEAFNESS.—Diminution or loss of hearing. It may result from hardened ear-wax, inflammation, paralysis, or mechanical obstruction. Syringing the ear daily with warm or tepid water, with attention to all existing morbid conditions, is the remedial plan. Many cases of partial, and some cases of complete deafness, are cured by purifying the mass of blood of its viscid and biliary impurities.

DEATH, APPARENT.—Asphyxia.

DEATH, BLACK.—The plague of the fourteenth century was so termed.

DEBILITY.—Asthenia, Weakness. This is never a cause, but always an effect of disease. Authors undertake to distinguish between *real* and *apparent* debility; but the terms *exhaustion* and *prostration* are more appropriate, and less liable to mislead.

DEBORDEMENT.—A French word applied to diarrhœa with discharges of a biliary character. See Diarrhœa.

DECIDENTIA —Epilepsy.

DECLINE.—See Phthisis; also Tabes.

DEER'S TEARS.—Bezoar of the Deer.

DEFLUXION.—Catarrh.

DEFLUXUS DYSENTERICUS.—Dysentery.

DEGENERATION.—A change for the worse in the solids or fluids; also any morbid alteration of structure, as cancerous, fungous, tubercular, etc.

DELIQUIUM ANIMI.—Syncope, Fainting.

DELIRIUM.—This affection is always symptomatic. It is frequently so violent in putrid fevers as to be mistaken for inflammation of the brain. Cold applications to the head, and warm to the feet, are always in order.

DELIRIUM, SENILE.—Demented.

DELIRIUM TREMENS.—Drunkard's Delirium, Mania-a-Potu, Delirium Ebriosita, Phrenitis Potatorum. A kind of delirium peculiar to those who indulge in the excessive use of opium, tobacco, strong tea and coffee, and especially alcohol. It is attended with extreme agitation, sleeplessness, and incoherency or falsity of language. It often succeeds the sudden abstraction of the customary excitant.

Medical men have not yet agreed whether the narcotic or stimulative plan of treatment is the best. But both are wrong. The warm-bath, the prolonged tepid half-bath, the tepid dripping-sheet, and, when the feverishness of the system is considerable and the patient manageable, the wet-sheet pack, are the proper remedial appliances; to be repeated two, three, or more times a day, as necessary. The bowels should be freed with enemas of tepid water; the head kept cool with cold wet cloths, and the feet kept warm with hot bottles, or frequent hot foot-baths. Fomentations to the abdomen will often quiet the nervous restlessness, and induce the needed sleep.

DELUSION.—Hallucination.

DEMENTIA.—Imbecility, Incoherent Insanity. This term is, in legal parlance, synonymous with insanity. But, in a strict medical sense, it applies to a state of idiocy. Mania, melancholy, and other forms of insanity, often ultimate in Dementia Doting is called the dementia of the aged. Constipation, torpid liver, violent mental excitement, and narcotic drugs, are among the causes of dementia.

DEMONOMANIA.—Religious Insanity. A kind of madness in which the person conceives himself possessed of devils, and is in continual dread of malignant spirits, death, eternal torments, etc. Violent emotions of the religious organs, especially under the additional influence of nervous excitants, as tea and coffee, may occasion it. Indigestion, in persons of a highly nervous temperament and over-wrought moral organs, predisposes to the complaint. Agreeable society, change of scenery, and all the resources of mental hygiene, should be employed.

DENGUE.—Dingee, Dandy, Rheumatic Fever, Bucket Fever. A disease which appeared in 1827 and 1828, in the Southern States, and in the West Indies, has been designated by these and many other names. It was extremely violent, but not dangerous. It differs from ordinary typhoid fevers, only in being attended with pain in the joints and muscles of the limbs. The fever usually terminated in two or three days, with copious perspiration. Dengue is, no doubt, a form of acute rheumatism. The warm-bath, followed, when the whole surface becomes hot, with the wet-sheet pack, and wet cloths to the affected joints, are all the bathing appliances the case requires.

DENTITION.—Dentitis. Though dentition is a normal process, there are many disorderly complications connected with it to which the term *teething* is applied. The *Temporary*, or milk-teeth, usually appear in the following order: Central incisors from the sixth to the eighth month; lateral incisors, seventh to tenth; first molar, twelfth to fourteenth; canines, fifteenth to twentieth; second molar, twentieth to thirtieth. The *Permanent Teeth* appear: first molars, seventh year; central incisors, eighth; lateral incisors, ninth; first bicuspids, tenth; second bicuspids, eleventh; canines, twelfth; second molars, thirteenth.

During the first dentition, the child is subject to pain, irritation and inflammation of the gums, the result mostly of disordered stomachs and constipated bowels. In some cases, a free division of the distended gum will give instant relief. But if the alimentary canal is duly attended to, this operation will be unnecessary.

DEPRESSION.—Dejection, Feebleness.

DERANDENITIS.—Inflammation of the glands of the neck. Apply cold wet cloths, covered with dry.

DERANGEMENT.—Disorder, Insanity, Displacement.

DERIVATION.—Antilepsis, Antispasis, Revulsion, Counteraction, Counter-determination. DUNGLISON says: "When a center of fluxion is established in a part, for the purpose of abstracting the vital manifestations from some other, a *derivation* is operated." Prof. PAYNE expresses the same idea much more lucidly: "We do but cure one disease by producing another." If the patient has apoplexy in the head, and the physician gives a drastic purgative, to produce diarrhœa in the bowels, the practice would be derivative—a misnomer, by the way, for the drug disease of the bowels does not *derive* its malady from the brain, but from the *medicine*.

DERMALGIA, DERMATALGIA.—Neuralgia of the nerves of the skin. It is always symptomatic. Treat the primary malady, whatever that may be.

DERMATITIS, DERMITIS.—Inflammation of the skin. See Erysipelas.

DERONCUS.—See Bronchocele.

DESMITIS.—Inflammation of Ligaments. It is a rheumatic affection.

DESQUAMATION.—Moulting. Exfoliation or separation of the epidermis or scarf-skin, in the form of scales. It is a common consequence of eruptive fevers, as scarlatina, measles, erysipelas, etc.

DESUDATIO.—Mucksweat. A profuse sweating, with an eruption of small pimples, similar to millet seeds. Children, who are not kept clean, are very subject to it. Tepid ablutions will remove it.

DETERMINATION.—"Rush of Blood." Increased or preternatural direction of blood and nervous energy to a part or organ. The remedy is *counter-determination*, that is, such appliance as will correct the abnormally disproportionate action and restore the balance of circulation. Thus, in apoplexy, we make cold applications to the head and warm to the feet; in inflammatory fever, we apply cold to the whole surface; in low typhoid fevers, warmth to the whole surface; in diptheria, croup, putrid sore throat, etc., cold to the throat and warmth to the extremities, while the surface is treated with warm, tepid or cool applications, according to its temperature. It is an important rule in Hygienic practice, that no powerful shock must be made upon the system, as with a douche, plunge, wet-sheet pack, shower, etc., when there is strong local determination, or much congestion of any important internal organ—the brain, lungs, liver, kidney, uterus etc.

DIABETES.— Urinary Diarrhœa, Excessive Discharge of Urine. It is attended with great thirst and progressive emaciation. In some cases the urine is saccharine, constituting the variety called *Diabetis Mellitys*. The function of the skin is exceedingly torpid, and the nutritive organs are all more or less deranged.

The main indication is to restore the action of the skin. Hot, warm, or tepid bathing should be resorted to daily, according to the condition of the superficial circulation. Usually the hot-bath, for five to ten minutes, followed by the tepid ablution, and this by dry, hand or towel rubbing, is one of the best of the bathing appliances. The vapor-bath is also excellent. The dry rubbing-sheet may be used advantageously once or twice a day, in a warm room. Local baths are of little use, and, if too cold, or too frequent, decidedly injurious. It is important to promote the respiratory functions as much as possible, in all possible ways. Gentle exercise in the open air, riding, light gymnastics, etc., are applicable to this indication. In the matter of diet, it only need be said that the more simple and plain it is the better. Sugar, milk, and grease, are especially objectionable. DUNGLISON says, "all the remedies which have been tried have usually been found inefficient." We have, however, cured many cases, and, indeed, all that we have treated Hygienically.

DIAPEDESIS.—Sweating of the Blood. Transudation of the blood, in the form of dew, at the surface of the skin, or of any membrane.

DIAPHORESIS.—Cutaneous Evacuation. Diaphoretic medicines, violent exertion, and many other causes, induce a morbidly increased excretion from the skin. The cure consists in removing the cause. Fevers, when attended with constant sweating, have been termed, not inappropriately, *Diaphoretic Fevers*.

DIAPHRAGMALGIA.—Pain in the Diaphragm.

DIAPHRAGMITIS.—Inflammation of the Diaphragm, Paraphrenitis. It cannot be, and need not be, distinguished from Pneumonitis, which see.

DIAPYEMIA.—Empyema, Suppuration.

DIARÆMIA.—A thin and putrescent condition of the blood, so that it transudes through the coats of the vessels into the cavities. It sometimes occurs in putrid fevers.

DIARRHŒA.—Looseness, Alvine Flux, Purging, Catharsis, Enterorrhœa, Intestinal Catarrh.—The chief varieties of this disease are distinguished by the character of the discharges, as *bilious, serous, chylous, mucous, diptheritic, fecal,* etc. They are all caused by the presence of irritating matter, accumulated feces, inflammation, or obstruction in some one or more of the depurating organs, so that there is a preternatural determination in the bowels.

After the intestinal tract has been well cleansed, with tepid enemas, if necessary, the warm hip-bath, or fomentations to the abdomen, will relieve the griping pain, and arrest the discharges. Small enemas of cold water, after each discharge, are advisable, in obstinate cases; also the wet-girdle, well covered with dry flannel. Exercising the respiratory apparatus, by means of deep, full inspirations and expirations, will often arrest the most aggravated forms of diarrhœa.

What is called *tubular diarrhœa* in medical books, is attended with a diptheritic excretion, which often hardens, and is expelled in fragments. These have been sometimes mistaken for cast-off portions of the mucous membrane. This is an obstinate, though not dangerous, malady, and can only be cured by a very strict dietary, in connection with such bathing appliances as tend to invigorate the skin and restore the digestive powers.

DIARRHŒA, HECTICA.—This term has been applied to a very fatal form of diarrhœa which prevails among the native inhabitants of India.

DIATHESIS.—State of the Body. In febrile diseases, there are two diathesis. The *high* and the *low*, entonic and atonic, etc. Inflammatory fever is always entonic, while typhoid and all other fevers are atonic. The term also applies to peculiar morbid conditions of chronic diseases, as *cancerous, scrofulous, scorbutic, arthritic, calculous, hemorrhagic, bilious,* etc.

DICHOPHYIA.—An affection of the hairs, in which they split and grow forked.

DIGITALATION.—I coin this word to express the disease induced by the medicinal employment of digitalis. It is known by slow, feeble pulse, coldness of the surface, dimness of sight, vertigo, and, when large doses have been given, delirium, vomiting, purging, hiccough, convulsions, and death. It has been extolled as a specific for consumption. "Why the drug is called digitalis," said an eminent medical professor, "I cannot imagine, unless it be that it points to the grave."

DINGEE.—Dengue.

DINOMANIA.—See Tarantismus.

DINUS.—Dizziness, Vertigo. A symptom in many diseases.

DIPTHERIA.—Diptherita, Diptheritis, Pellicular Inflammation. An inflammatory affection of the mucous membrane, and sometimes of the skin, in which there is a fibrinous excretion, forming, when concreted on the surface, a membraneous coating, termed *false membrane.* It affects most frequently the mouth, throat, nose, and upper part of the windpipe, though it may extend even into the bronchial ramifications.

The excretion should be arrested as promptly as possible, by cold applications to the throat, frequent sips of the coldest water, and bits of ice held and allowed to melt in the mouth. This treatment must be persevered in until the preternatural heat is permanently relieved. Meanwhile, the system must be treated according to the development of the febrile symptoms. When the whole surface is hot and dry, and the constitution not feeble nor scrofulous, the wet-sheet pack is advisable; when the external heat is less, the tepid ablution is preferable; if the superficial heat is unequal, the warm-bath should be employed. The feet must at all times be kept warm, and ventilation carefully attended to. When, in the later stage, there is suffocative respiration, and difficult expectoration, fomentations to the chest and abdomen, with frequent sips of warm water, should be employed.

DɪPLOPɪA.—Double Vision. An affection of the sight, in which there are two distinct recognitions of one object. In some cases several objects are seen, when the malady is called *Suffusio Multiplicans.* The defect is in the visual axes, and is a case for the oculist.

DɪPLOSOMA.—This term has been applied to an entozoon which is sometimes expelled from the urinary bladder. It is several inches in length, and doubled upon itself so as to appear like two worms tied together at their heads.

DɪPSOMANɪA.—Thirst Mania. An insatiable desire for intoxicating drinks. The term is sometimes applied to habitual drunkenness, and to delirium tremens.

DɪPSOSɪS.—Morbid Thirst. Excessive or impaired desire for drink: It is always symptomatic.

DɪSCRETE.—Separate, Distinct. This term is applied to the spots or pustules of measles, small-pox, and other exanthems, when they are separated from each other. When they run or blend together, they are termed *confluent. Discrete* eruptions always indicate the milder forms of eruptive fevers, while the *confluent* denote the malignant or extremely putrid cases.

DɪSEASE.—Nosos, Morbus, Pathos, Malady, Sickness, Complaint, Distemper, Disorder, Affection, Indisposition. The medical profession has always labored under a strange delusion with regard to the nature or essence of disease; and the authors are perpetually confounding diseases with their causes. Disease is remedial effort—the veritable "*vis medicatrix naturæ*" itself. Yet the medical profession have ever regarded it, and still do regard it, as a mysterious entity; an incomprehensible something at war with the vital powers. When they discover the very simple truth that disease is vital action in relation to things abnormal—a defensive struggle, an effort to purify the system of morbific materials, and repair the damages—there will be a speedy revolution in medical science. And when the people can be made to understand this, they will no more think of taking poisons because they are sick, than they will think of taking them because they are well.

The following table, by Dr. C. J. B. WILLIAMS, presents, at a glance, the chief elements of structural diseases:

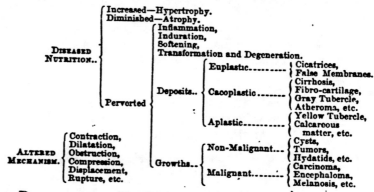

DISGORGEMENT.— Vomiting. Also the abstraction of fluid previously collected in a part. The opposite of *Engorgement*.

DISGUST.—Loathing, Aversion for Food. It exists in the early stages of many acute diseases, and is symptomatic, in some extreme cases, of indigestion.

DISLOCATION.—Luxation. The displacement of one or more bones of a joint.

DISORDER.—See Disease.

DISORGANIZATION.—An abnormal change in the structure of an organ or part.

DISPLACEMENT.—This term is applied to various malpositions of organs, and especially those of the uterus, which are technically termed *Prolapsus, Anteversion, Retroversion,* and *Inversion,* as the organ is depressed, inclined forward, tipped backward, or turned inside out. For a full explanation of these cases, see the author's works, "Uterine Diseases and Displacements," and "Pathology of the Reproductive Organs."

DISPOSITION.—This term is sometimes used in the sense of Diathesis, and sometimes Predisposition, which see.

DISSOLUTION.—This word is sometimes employed to indicate an impoverished state of the blood, not amounting to putrefaction.

DISTEMPER.—See Disease.

DISTOMA HEPATICUM.—Gourd Worm, Fluke, Liver Fluke, Fasciola Hepatica. An obovate, flat worm about an inch in length, and nearly as broad. It is sometimes found in the human gall-bladder, whence it occasionally passes through the bile-ducts into the intestinal canal. It is one of the most common kinds of worms which infest the livers of domestic animals, especially those which are stye or stall-fed. The filthy enclosures and the foul food are the chief causes; and cleanliness, "natural food" and proper exercise, are the appropriate remedies.

DISTORTION.—Preternatural curvature of the bony structure. It is sometimes applied to morbidly contracted muscles, as in Squinting. Distorted spines seem to be, like consumption, scrofula, dyspepsia, constipation, etc., one of the increasing maladies of these degenerate days. They require gymnastic and "Movement" exercises, and machinery, under the direction of a competent physician.

DISTRIX.—An affection in which the hairs of the scalp become slender, and split at their extremities. The excessive use of salt, night work, and various other causes, may induce it. The hair should be cut short, the scalp wet, morning and evening, with cold water, and occasionally shampooed.

DITRACHYCERAS.—An intestinal entozoön, of a fawn color, three to five lines in length, with an oval head, furnished anteriorly with a bifurcated, rugous horn. See Worms.

DIURESIS.—Copious urinary excretion. Tea, coffee, gin, and other diuretic beverages or medicines, may occasion it. It may also result from deficient action of the skin. Dry diet, water-drinking only to the extent of actual thirst, and tepid ablutions with abundant friction of the skin, dry rubbing, etc., are the remedies.

DIZZINESS.—See Vertigo.

DOG-CHOAK.—See Cynanche.

DOLOR.—Pain—not a disease, but an indication of disease. Every organ and structure, when diseased, has its peculiar morbid feeling, or pain, as each part, in health, has its own normal feeling, or sensation. Were it not for the beneficent provision of pain, the mind could never come to the assistance of the vital organism in its difficulties and derangements.

DORMITATIO.—See Somnolency.

DOTAGE.—See Dementia.

DOTHIEN.—See Furunculus.

DOTHIENTERIA, DOTHIENTERITIS.—Inflammation and ulceration of the glands or follicles of PEYER and BRUNNER, and which have been very absurdly regarded as the essence, seat, or cause of typhus and typhoid fevers. They are merely an indicant, not an "essence" of these diseases.

DOUBLE HEARING.—Sounds heard doubly, and in different tones or keys, because the action of the ears is unaccordant.

DRACUNCULUS.—Muscular Hair Worm, Guinea Worm, Threadworm. A variety of worms, common to parts of India and Africa. When small, they may pass through the pores of the skin, into the areolar tissue between the muscles, where they occasion a tumor, like a boil, which suppurates, when the worm emerges. "Its head may then be seized, and the animal be cautiously rolled round a small cylinder of linen or other substance, and thus gently withdrawn without breaking it."

It is well to remark that, all authors do not credit this process of cure, and some deny that the reported cases of Dracunculus, are really worms at all.

DRIVELLING.—See Slavering.

DROP.—See Gutta.

DROPPED HANDS.—Hand Drop, Wrist Drop. A popular term for paralysis of the hand, occasioned by lead.

DROPSY.—Hydrops. An accumulation of watery fluid in the cavities or areolar tissue. There are several varieties which are treated of under their respective heads, as Anasarca, Ascites, Hydrocephalus, Hydrothorax, Hydrometra, Hydropthalmia, etc.

DRUG DISEASE.—Drugalgia, Drugitis, Drugodynia, Drugania Druggery, Drugopathy, Poisonopathy. When it is considered that, a majority of all chronic maladies extant, are nothing more nor less than drug diseases, and that as many people are sent to their graves prematurely by drug medicines, as by all other causes combined, we need not wonder at the strong expression of an earnest health reformer who pronounced the civilized world to be "doctor-cursed and drug-damned."

DRUNKENNESS.—Temulentia, Intoxication, Ebrietas, Delirium, Mania, Hallucination; or Insensibility induced by alcoholic liquors. Drunkenness requires the same treatment as apoplexy.

DUMBNESS.—Mutitas, Speechlessness, inability to articulate. When congenital, and arising from deafness, the subjects of it are called, *Deaf-Dumb.*

DUNGA.—See Dengue.

DUODENITIS.—Inflammation of the duodenum, or upper portion of the intestinal tube. Dyspeptics, especially those who have deranged livers with an excretion of acrid bile, are very liable to it in a chronic form. It is characterized by a sense of "goneness," gnawing, sinking, or burning just below the pit of the stomach, furred tongue, bad taste, and tenderness in the epigastric region. Eating will at any time relieve it for the time. Fomentations and the wet-girdle, with simple, solid food, are the special remedial appliances; meanwhile the general health, and the morbid condition of the liver and digestive organs should be attended to.

DYNAMIC DISEASES.—In contradistinction to *organic diseases,* which are attended with structural lesions, dynamic diseases are those which necessarily involve only functional diseases. Fevers are dynamic or functional diseases, while aneurisms, cancers, etc., are structural, organic diseases.

DYSÆMIA.—A morbid condition of the blood. Strictly speaking, this is more or less the case in every disease.

DYSÆSTHESIA.—Diminution, or loss of sensation.

DYSCRASIA.—Dyscrasy, Dysthetica. A bad habit of body. See cachexia.

DYSENTERY.—Bloody Flux, Colitis, Colomitis, Colo-Rectitis. Inflammation of the mucous membrane of the large intestines, characterized by fever, mucus, or bloody discharges, with violent tormina and tenesmus. DUNGLISON says, "the fever is more or less inflammatory." This is a sad mistake, and leads to grave errors in practice. The local affection is always inflammatory, but the fever is always typhoid. In cases of extreme putridity, the disease is called *Malignant Dysentery*. Dysentery is always acute. What is called *chronic dysentery* is merely severe diarrhœa.

The first indication in the treatment is to reduce the excessive heat and pain in the abdomen, by means of cold wet cloths, frequently changed. After this has been accomplished, the bowels should be freely moved, and then if the pain and griping continue, fomentations should be applied to the abdomen, to be followed by cold and wet cloths covered with dry. The general bathing must be regulated by the degree of external heat. If the whole surface is hot and dry, the wet sheet should be employed; if the superficial heat is very unequal, the warm bath is appropriate; if equal and moderate, tepid ablutions are preferable. Though a very distressing malady, under proper treatment, it is not at all dangerous.

DYSLOCHIA.—Diminution or suppression of the lochial discharge. Warm hip-baths, hot foot-baths, and fomentations will relieve the difficulty.

DYSMENORRHŒA.—Painful Menstruation. The menstrual fluid is passed with difficulty, and not unfrequently with excruciating pain, of a "bearing-down" kind.

There is more or less of a membraneous or diptheritic formation on the mucous membrane of the uterus, which is expelled in fragments, as in croup, diphtheria, tubular diarrhœa, and catarrh of the bladder. No disease, not excepting cancer, plague, cholera, consumption, diabetis, etc., has been treated with less success, confessedly, by the medical profession than this; and for no ill that flesh is heir to, have mortals been more unmercifully and ruinously bled, blistered, cauterized, salivated, and narcotized.

The disease is one of chronic inflammation, and should be treated accordingly, with tepid hip-baths, the wet-girdle, hot-and-cold foot-baths, etc. But it is always connected with, and the consequence of, some morbid condition of the general system, which must be remedied, or no cure can be permanent. Out-door exercise—all the patient can take without fatigue, abdominal manipulations, and the light gymnastics, are useful. For general bathing, the tepid ablution or dripping sheet is usually preferable. While there is comparatively a good degree of external circulation, the wet-sheet pack should be employed once or twice a week. To relieve the pain during or preceding the menstrual flux, the hot-bath and abdominal fomentations are often necessary. Warm vaginal injections may be also employed for this purpose. Milk, butter, cheese, sugar and salt should be excluded from the dietary, as should puddings, mushes, broths, soups, and all preparations of starch and eggs.

DYSODIA.—Fetid emanations from the mouth, nose, lungs, stomach, axillæ, groins, etc. They indicate bad blood, and foul secretions, imperfect depuration, retained fecal matters, etc. Judicious bathing, and a proper dietary, with sufficient exercise in the open air, will remove them.

DYSOPIA.—Difficulty of seeing.

DYSOPIA DISSITORUM.—See Myopia.

DYSOPIA LATERALIS.—Sight-askew, Skew-Sight. A morbid condition of the eye in which an object can only be recognized accurately when placed obliquely. It is generally caused by some opacity of the cornea.

DYOSMIA.—Diminution of smell. It may be the effect of chronic inflammation, or of irritant drugs.

DYSPEPSIA.—Difficulty of Digestion, Indigestion, Anorexia, Apepsia, Gastroataxia.

The symptoms of Dyspepsia are as numerous as are morbid sensations; for the whole catalogue of human maladies scarcely furnishes a sign of bodily derangement, or of mental distress, which is not found in some form or stage of the disease under consideration. The more prominent and uniform symptoms are, capricious appetite, irregular action of the bowels, and sense of weight or pain after meals. Heartburn, acrid eructations, flatulence, duodenitis, throbbing, fluttering, or palpitation of the heart, etc., are common accompaniments.

As bad living, and especially unwholesome food, are the prominent causes, a correct dietary should be the leading feature in the process of cure. And the rule happens to be exceedingly simple and eminently practicable. Bread made of unbolted meal and pure water, with no admixture of grease, sugar, salt, acids, or alkalies, with good ripe fruits, should be the principal food. Vegetables may be used in moderation, but only one or two kinds at a meal. Two meals a day are generally better than three. It is of the first importance that the patient eat very slowly, and swallow nothing without thorough mastication. This rule applies with still more emphasis in the use of fruit. Slop-food, mushes, puddings, etc., should be eschewed. The exercises should be frequent and varied, but not very fatiguing. Those which exercise the respiratory and abdominal muscles should be most resorted to, as walking on uneven ground, the light gymnastics, rowing, horse-back riding, moderate dancing, etc. "Early to bed and early to rise," is an invaluable adage for the dyspeptic. Indeed abundant sleep is as important as proper food. All exciting or vexing brain-labor should be as much as possible avoided. Vocal gymnastics, reading aloud, singing, declamation, etc., are as useful to the dyspeptic as to the incipient consumptive. In many cases the abdominal muscles are extremely enfeebled and inactive, and whether rigid or relaxed, can be greatly benefitted by the "Swedish Movements."

Dyspeptics should carefully avoid *watching their own sensations and noting their ever-changing symptoms*, as the manner of some is. Nothing can be more pernicious. They should study their cases and seek information until satisfied what the proper plan is, then "go ahead," and trust to Providence and their own recuperative energies.

DYSPHAGIA.—Difficulty of Deglutition. It may be caused by spasm, or paralysis of the œsophagus, or a thickening of its mucous membrane in consequence of chronic inflammation. The treatment must have reference to these conditions. In the latter case everything of a heating or irritant nature must be excluded from the dietary, or the disease may be aggravated until swallowing is impossible, and starvation be the result.

DYSPHAGIA CONSTRICTA.—Stricture of the Œsophagus. When the thickened mucous membrane becomes permanently indurated the only remedy is the bougie.

DYSPHONIA.—Imperfect or depraved voice. The *Aphonia* of some authors.

DYSPNŒA.—Pseudo-Asthma, Anhelation, Short Breath, Difficulty of Breathing. This affection is symptomatic of asthma, pneumonia, hydrothorax, enlargement of the liver, empyema, phthisis, and various other maladies.

DYSTHESIA.—Morbid Habit. See Cachexia.

DYSTHETICA.—Morbid condition of the blood. See Plethora.

DYSTŒCHIASIS. — Irregular position of the eye-lashes. Sometimes they incline inward and irritate the eyelids, in which case they should be removed.

DYSURIA.—Difficult Urination. It is symptomatic of gonorrhœa, stricture, gravel, etc., and is the first degree of retention of the urine. It may generally be relieved by warm or tepid bathing.

EBRIETAS, EBRIOSITAS,—Temulentia. See Drunkenness.

ECCHYMOMA.—Ecchymosis, Livor Sanguinis, Hypocœmia. A livid, black, or yellow blotch produced by blood effused into the areolar tissue from a contusion. Cold water will facilitate the absorption of the effused matter. Spontaneous effusions occurring in disease or after death are called *suggillations*.

ECHINOPHTHALMIA.—Inflammation of the eyelids in which the cilia project like the quills of the porcupine.

ECLAMPSIA.—Convulsion.

ECPHLOGOSIS.—Inflammation.

ECPHLYSIS.—See Herpes.

ECPHRONIA.—Insanity.

ECPHYMA.—Excrescence, Tumor.

ECPYEMA, ECPYESIS.—Abscess, Pustule.

ECSTASIS.—Ecstacy, Trance, Spurious Catalepsy.

ECTHYMA.—Ecpyesis, Scabies Vera. A cutaneous eruption characterized by large, round pustules, distinct, with an indurated and highly inflamed base. The wet-sheet pack should be employed daily, and the patient restricted to a plain and abstemious diet.

ECTOPIA.—Displacement, Laxation.

ECTOZOA.—Lice and other parasitic animals which infest the skin.

ECTROPION.—Eversion of the eyelids. It may generally be remedied by removing a portion of the conjunctiva.

ECZEMA.—Humid Tetter, Running Scall, Heat Eruption. An eruption of small vesicles on various parts of the skin. The wet-sheet pack, or tepid ablutions, and a strict diet are advisable.

ECZEMA MERCURIALE.—Erythema Mercuriale, Eczema Rubrum, Hydrargyriosis, Morbus Mercurialis. Mercurial Leprosy. A variety of Eczema caused by mercurial medicines. Patients who are strongly infected with the mercurial poison do not bear very cold baths with advantage. A warm bath daily, followed by the tepid ablution, and the wet-sheet pack once or twice a week, can almost always be employed beneficially. Salt, sugar, milk and all greasy things should be excluded from the dietary. Where the skin is abraded or ulcers appear, the part should be covered and the cavity filled with fine flour daily.

ECZEMA OF THE FACE.—See Porrigo Larvalis.

ECZEMA IMPETIGINODES.—Gall Itch, Grocers' Itch. This is produced by the irritation of sugar.

ECZEMA OF THE HAIRY SCALP.—This differs from *Porrigo* and *Tinea*, in the eruption being vesicular instead of pustular. The discharge is very profuse, and in drying into crusts mats the hair into separate tufts. It is often complicated with scrofulous swellings or ulcers. A variety of this disease has been called *Asbestos Scall*.

ECZEMATOSES.—A term applied to a group of cutaneous diseases, of which there are many subdivisions.

EDEMATOUS.—See Œdematous.

EDENTULOUS.—Toothlessness. See a good Dentist.

EFFLORATIO.—See Exanthem.

EFFLORESCENCE.—Cutaneous Blush. The term is sometimes employed as synonymous with exanthem.

EFFUSION.—The passing of blood or any other fluid into the cavities of the body, or into the areolar tissue. The excretion of coagulable lymph, on membraneous surfaces, during the process of inflammation, is called effusion; as is also the pouring out of serum. Effusion into the areolar membrane is more frequently termed *infiltration*.

EGREGORSIS. — Vigilantia, Watchfulness. See Sleeplessness.

ELCOSIS.—Ulceration. A deep ulcer of the cornea.

ELEPHANTIASIS.—Barbadoes Leg, Bucnemia Tropica, Cochin Leg, Lepra Arabum, Mal Rouge de Cayenne, Pellagra. Various affections of the people of Barbadoes, India, Arabia, Cayenne, Greece, Italy and Java, have been described as Elephantiasis. Generally the term is applied to a condition in which the skin becomes thick, rugous, tuberculated, and insensible. In the Elephantiasis of the Antilles the leg is enormously swollen and misshapen; in the Indian and Arabian malady the tubercles are chiefly on the face and joints; the Cayenne and Greek disease resembles a variety of Leprosy, and is characterized by red and yellow spots on the forehead, ears, hands, loins, etc.; in the Italian the skin is wrinkled and scaly; and in the disease as it appears in Java, white tumors affect the toes and fingers, resembling scrofulous swellings.

In whatever form the disease appears, it indicates extreme depravity of blood, with great obstruction in, or torpor of, the whole excrementous system. Hence purification in all possible ways, is the sum and substance of the required treatment.

EMACIATION.—Leanness. This is not a disease, but an effect of disease: To obviate it we have only to restore the normal condition.

EMANSIO MENSIUM.—See Amenorrhœa.

EMESIS.—Vomiting, Puking. Tartarized Antimony, Ipecacuanha, Sulphate of Zinc, Sulphate of. Copper, Yellow Sulphate of Mercury, Sanguinaria Canadensis, and Lobelia, are the drugs most commonly employed *medicinally*, to produce the *disease*, Emesis. See Vomiting.

EMETO-CATHARSIS.—Vomiting and Purging. When occasioned by medicinal drugs it is called an *emeto-cathartic operation*, and when induced by other "morbid poisons," it is termed *cholera*. "What's in a name?"

EMPATHEMA.—Ungovernable passion.

EMPHLYSIS.—Ichorous Exanthem. An eruption of vesicular pimples, filled with a colorless but acrid fluid, and terminating in scurf or laminated scabs. Warm baths or tepid ablutions should be employed.

EMPHYMA.—Tumor.

EMPHYSEMA.—Pneumatosis, Flatulent Tumor, Inflation, Wind-Dropsy. An elastic, crepitant tumor occasioned by the introduction of air into the aréolar texture. It may result from injuries of the larynx, trachea or lungs, fractures of the ribs, or wounds penetrating the chest.

EMPHYSEMA ABDOMINIS.—See Tympanites:

EMPHYSEMA OF THE LUNGS.—The chest externally appears abnormally convex and prominent; the intercostal spaces are widened, but depressed; the inspiratory efforts are increased and expiration is laborious, wheezing, and prolonged. Rest and ventilation are the essential remedial conditions, aside from such surgery as the case may require.

EMPRESMA.—Inflammation.,

EMPROSTHOTONOS.—Tetanus Anticus. That form of Tetanus in which the body is bent forward. See Tetanus.

EMPYEMA.—Apostema Empyema. A collection of blood or pus in some cavity of the body. It is most frequently found in the cavity of the pleura, and is said to be one of the *terminations* of inflammation of the lungs or pleura. But as the inflammation seldom or never "terminates" at that time, it were better to say, one of the *consequences* of inflammation. When the collection is large the surgical operation of *parencentesis thoracis* is necessary to remove the collected matter.

EMPYESIS.—Pustular Exanthem. An eruption of pimples gradually filling with a purulent fluid, and terminating in thick scales, frequently leaving pits or scabs, as in small-pox.

EMPYOCELE.—Accumulation of pus in the Scrotum. The tumor should be opened.

ENANTHESIS.—Rash Exanthem.

ENANTHESIS ROSALIA.—A term including *Scarlatina* and *Urticuria*, which see.

ENCANTHIS.—Any morbid growth in the inner angle of the eye. Commonly applied to a tumefaction or degeneration of the *caruncula lachrymalis.* It may be cured by repeated refrigerations or freezings, and attention to the general health.

ENCANTHIS BENIGNA.—Simple excrescence of the caruncula. It yields to cold applications, or mild caustics.

ENCANTHIS FUNGOSA.—Morbid growths of the lachrymal caruncle.   Refrigeration and cauterization are the remedies.

ENCANTHIS INFLAMMATORY,—Inflammation of the caruncle. It only requires cold applications.

ENCANTHIS MALIGNA.—A cancerous affection of the gland. It should be removed at once by the refrigerating and cauterizing process.

ENCAUSIS.—Moxibustion, Encauma. See Burn.

ENCEPHALALGIA.—Hydrocephalus Internus.

ENCEPHALITIS.—Cephalitis, Phrenitis, Inflammation of the Brain. See Cephalitis.

6

ENCEPHALOCELE.—Fungus Cerebri, Hernia of the Brain. It may be congenital or accidental, and dependent on tardy ossification of the fontanelles, or loss of substance in the bones of the skull. When the tumor is small, it may be remedied by gentle pressure on the protruded portion of the brain. In other cases it is fatal.

ENCEPHALOID.—Scirrhous and cancerous tumors are so called, when they resemble the medullary substance of the brain. They are also called *Medullary*.

ENCYSTED.—Pouched, Saccated, Sacculated. A term applied to tumors whose contents are enclosed in a cyst, or membraneous sac. They are movable and often elastic. The remedy is excision, or puncture.

ENDEMIC.—Diseases are called endemic when they prevail in a given locality, or district, or neighborhood; *epidemic* when they extend over several districts or neighborhoods, and *sporadic* when they appear in isolated cases.

ENDOCARDITIS.—Inflammation of the internal membrane of the heart—the *endocardium*. It cannot be, and need not be distinguished from Carditis.

ENDOCOLITIS.—Dysentery.

ENDODONTITIS.—Inflammation of the lining membrane of a tooth. See Odontitis.

ENDO-ENTERITIS.—See Enteritis.

ENDOGASTRITIS. Inflammation of the lining membrane of the stomach. See Gastritis.

ENDOMETRITIS.—See Metritis.

ENICIA.—Synochus, Inflammatory Fever.

ENERVATION.—Debility, Weakness.

ENGLISH DISEASE.—Rachitis.

ENGORGEMENT.—Congestion. Disproportionate accumulation of blood in the vessels of a part.

ENOSTOSIS.—A morbid growth of bone inwards—the opposite of Exostosis.

ENTASIA.—Tonic spasm, as Cramp, Tetanus, etc.

ENTERALGIA.—Enterodynia, Colic.

ENTERITIS.—Ileo-Colitis, Enteralgia acuta. Inflammation of the intestines. The essential symptoms are, violent pain, increased on pressure, with heat and swelling of the abdomen, and fever, which may be either of the inflammatory or typhoid diathesis. The distinction of enteritis into the *sero* and *muco* varieties, as the serous or mucous coat is the seat of it, is simply absurd. It is enough for all practical purposes, and is all that can be known without a post-mortem examination, to know that the bowels are in a state of inflammation.

The morbid heat of the abdomen must be subdued by cold applications, which can usually be accomplished in a few hours, after which the bowels should be freely moved with tepid enemas. Cool but not very cold water may be drank *ad libitum*. The whole surface must be sponged with tepid water two or three times a day, and if the superficial heat is very great, the wet-sheet-pack should be employed daily. In the low, or typhoid cases, care must be taken to keep the circulation balanced, and the extremities warm.

ENTEROCELE.—Abdominal hernia, containing only a portion of intestine.

ENTEROCYSTOCELE.—Hernia formed by the bladder and a portion of intestine.

ENTERO-EPIPLOCELE.—Hernia formed by intestine and omentum.

ENTERO-EPIPLOMPHALUS.—Umbilical hernia, containing intestine and omentum.

ENTERO-HYDROCELE.—Intestinal hernia, complicated with hydrocele.

ENTERO-HYDROMPHALUS.—Umbilical hernia, in which the sac contains intestine and serum.

ENTERO-ISCHIOCELE.—Ischiatic hernia, formed of intestine.

ENTEROLITHUS.—Calculi of the stomach and intestines. Bezoar, Scybula. See Calculi.

ENTERO-MEROCELE.—Crural hernia, formed of intestine.

ENTERO-MESENTERIC FEVER.—An awkward term for the nervous form of typhus fever.

ENTEROZOA.—Worms.

ENTHELMINTHES.—Worms.

ENTHEOMANIA.—See Demonomania.

ENTONIC.—Strong determination to the surface, as in high fevers; the opposite of *atonic*. Medical men, almost universally, recognize the principle of depletion in entonic, and stimulation in atonic diathesis. But both practices are wrong. In the one case, the determination is too violent *to* the surface, and the other, too violent *from* the surface. The indication is not to reduce the blood, nor poison it, but simply to *balance the circulation*. Were this principle recognized, thousands of lives would be saved annually.

ENTOPARASITES.—Worms.

ENTOPHTHALMIA.—Inflammation of the interior of the eye. See Opthalmia.

ENTOXISMUS.—Poisoning. The treatment of disease, according to the drug system, is, from beginning to end, a toxicological process. Says PROFESSOR PAINE, in his "Institutes of Medicine," "We do but cure one disease by producing another."

ENTOZOA, ENTOZOAIRES.—Worms.

ENTROPION, ENTROPIUM.—Trichiasis. Inversion of the eyelids, by means of which the eyelashes irritate and inflame the eye. It may be remedied by cutting out a portion of the skin.

ENURESIS.—Urorrhœa, Incontinence of Urine, Involuntary urination. It may be due to paralysis, atony, over-distention, calculi, morbid irritability, or pressure from a tumor or displaced uterus. The treatment may be adapted to the cause; and when this cannot be removed, the urethra must be compressed by appropriate instruments, or what is better, a urinal may be constantly worn.

EPHELIDES.—Freckles, Sunburn. This term includes the yellow discolorations which appear on persons of a fair skin, the brown patches which arise from exposure to the sun, and the large dusky patches which occur on parts of the body covered with the clothing.

EPHEMERA.—One Day Fever.

EPHIDROSIS.—Profuse sweating. It is symptomatic in many low fevers and states of debility.

EPIDEMIC, EPIDEMY.—A disease which prevails over a large tract of country, or in several districts.

EPIGASTROCELE.—Gastrocele, Hernia formed by the stomach.

EPIGLOTTITIS.—Inflammation of the glottis. See Laryngitis.

EPILEPSY.—Falling sickness. The convulsive paroxysms are characterized by loss of sensation and voluntary motion, distortion of the eyes and face, foaming at the mouth, and frequently sterterous breathing. The fit lasts from a few seconds to several minutes. In some cases the spasms are preceded by the sensation of cold vapor, termed *Aura Epileptica*. Furious mania sometimes succeeds a paroxysm, which is termed *Mania Epileptica*, or *Epileptic Delirium*.

Epileptic spasms may arise from structural lesions of the brain or spinal marrow, or from functional derangements, more especially obstructions or irritations in the alimentary canal. The former class of cases are generally incurable; the latter are mostly curable. Epileptic spasms are not unfrequently owing to nervous exhaustion, consequent on dissipation or debauchery of some kind. Over-exertion, mental excitement, an indigestible meal, and sexual indulgence are common exciting causes.

In the treatment little can be done during the paroxysm except to prevent the patient from injuring himself. During the intervals a rigidly simple and rather abstemious dietary must be adopted. The bathing appliances must be carefully adapted to the circumstances of each case. The tepid dripping-sheet, or half bath can almost always be taken once a day with advantage. The best time is on rising in the morning. The hip-bath—75° to 85°—may be taken for ten minutes once or twice daily, say at 10 A. M., and 5 P. M., and when there is tendency to coldness of the feet, or heat in the head, the hot-and-cold foot-bath should be taken at bedtime. The wet-sheet pack, once or twice a week is advisable for those who have an active external circulation. As there is almost always torpor of the abdominal viscera with constipation, abdominal manipulations, with "movements," are highly serviceable. Enemas of tepid water should be employed when the bowels do not incline to act without. When the patient is subject to much heat in the head, with a tendency to feverishness and a flushed face, the forehead and top-head should be wet with cold water two or three times a day, and on retiring at night; but I protest against the wet head-cap in such cases as its effect is to induce determination to the head, whereas the indication of cure is just the contrary. It may be necessary to persevere in this plan for weeks, and sometimes for months, before the cure is obtained.

EPIPHORA.—Weeping, watery eye. A constant and involuntary flow of tears upon the cheek. It is commonly owing to an obstruction of the lachrymal passages so that the tears cannot pass into the nasal duct. In some cases of irritation and inflammation the complaint is due to the excessive excretion. The remedial plan is, to remove the inflammation and open the obstructed passage, by a probe, if necessary.

EPIPLOCELE.—Omental Hernia.

EPISTAXIS—Bleeding at the nose. It occurs most frequently at the period of puberty, when, unless the depurating organs are in good working order there is a special tendency to plethora. Plain food, free bowels, and an active skin, are sure preventives, except when the affection results from mechanical injuries.

Many expedients have been resorted to successfully to arrest the hemorrhage. Cold water applied to the head and nasal passages, with hot foot-baths often succeed. When the whole body is hot and feverish, a cold ablution or half-bath will succeed. In severe cases the bowels should be freely moved with enemas of tepid water. When the bleeding is excessive the nostrils should be plugged with lint or soft sponge. Nasal hemorrhage has often been arrested by compressing the nostril with the finger, while the patient stands with the head elevated and raises the corresponding arm perpendicularly.

EPIZOA.—Parasitic animals, which infest the surface.

EPIZOOTIA.—Epidemic. Usually applied to diseases of cattle in the sense that epidemic is to diseases of human beings.

EPOSTOMA, EPOSTOSIS.—See Exostosis.

EPULIS.—An excrescence on the gum, sometimes becoming cancerous. It should be removed with caustic.

EQUINIA.—Glanders. It affects chiefly the horse, the ass, and the mule, and from them the causes may be communicated to man. It is a pustular and contagious exanthem like small-pox. The disease closely resembles the plague in man. Veterinary surgeons describe two varieties, one of which is attended with a profuse discharge from the nostrils, with eruptions of small suppurating tumors, and symptoms of gangrene in various parts, and the other, appearing in the shape of small tumors about the lips, face, neck, etc. The latter form is called *Farcy Glanders*. Both forms occasionally co-exist. Each is attended with malignant fever; or rather, the disease is always malignant.

An equable, mild temperature, pure air, tepid ablutions followed by friction with a hair brush, and thin water gruel, provided the animal can be made to drink it, constitute the remedial plan.

ERETHISM.—Orgasm. Augmentation of vital phenomena, in any organ or tissue. Medical authors generally mistake *abnormal* vital manifestations for augmented or increased vitality, and so bleed, antiphlogisticate, reduce, and *antivitalize* their *erethismatic* patients, and with most disastrous results. The term is often applied to parts in a condition of irritation or inflammation.

ERETHISMUS.—Erethism, Irritation. *Mercurial erethismus* is characterized by great depression of strength; anxiety about the præcordia; irregular action of the heart; frequent sighing; tremors; small, quick, sometimes intermittent pulse; occasional vomiting; pale, contracted countenance, and sense of coldness. In this state any sudden exertion may prove fatal.

All that can be done remedially, is, to keep the patient as quiet as possible; let him drink tepid or warm water in small drafts, as often as he can without provoking nausea, and sponge the surface two or three times a day, with tepid or warm water.

The preparations of antimony, gold, iron, iodine, etc., when used medicinally, often induce *erethismus* or *mineral fever*, quite as fatal, though more obscure in the *phenomena* of poisoning. The patient may die of the *drug inflammation*, without manifesting any symptoms which would be recognized by the medical attendant, as indicating a poisonous or dangerous effect of the *remedy*.

ERGOTISM.—Poisoning by Ergot. The morbid condition or disease occasioned by *Ergot* or *Spurred Rye*, whether taken accidentally, or administered medicinally. The prominent symptoms are, vertigo, numbness of the hands and feet, spasms, followed, in extreme cases, by gangrene and death. Ergot is frequently employed as a parturifacient, to intensify uterine contractions in protracted labors, on the absurd theory that, it has a "special affinity" to act on the muscular structure of the gravid uterus. But it is extremely liable to occasion uterine hemorrhage, convulsions, hour-glass contractions, etc., in the mother, and the death or permanent decrepitude of the child.

As in all cases of narcotic poisoning, the remedial plan for Ergotism is, perfect quiet; cold applications to the head, and warm to the feet; tepid ablutions; an elevated position of the head, and ample ventilation.

EROMANIA—EROTOMANIA.—Erotic Passion, Melancholy, Delirium, or ungovernable Sexual Passion, arising from sexual excitement or disappointment. See Nymphomania and Satyriasis.

ERRATIC.—Wandering, Irregular. Rheumatic affections, Agues, Menstrual disorders, etc., are so termed when they manifest no regular form or type.

ERUCTATION.—Belching; a dyspeptic symptom. Dry, solid food will relieve it.

ERUPTION.—This term applies to rashes, vesicles, pustules, etc., which appear on the surface, and also to the sudden evacuation of any fluid, as serum, blood, or pus, from a canal or cavity. Several hundreds of cutaneous eruptions have been recognized by authors, and treated of as distinct diseases. All of them which are important, are mentioned in this work, both under the technical and their popular names.

ERUPTIVE.—Applied to fevers which are essentially accompanied with cutaneous eruptions. They are *Small-pox, Measles, Scarlatina, Erysipelas, Miliaria*, and *Plague*, constituting the *Exanthems* of GOOD's "Study of Medicine."

ERYSIPELAS.—St. Anthony's Fire; superficial inflammation of the skin, with general fever, tension, redness and swelling of the part, and an acrid, burning heat. The redness disappears on pressure. In some cases of Erysipelas the fever is very mild, but in other forms it is extremely putrid and malignant, and liable to terminate in gangrene. There are no maladies in which mercurials are more freely prescribed, and do more extensive mischief, than the malignant fever of Erysipelas.

As the head and face are ordinarily most violently affected, they must be kept cool by means of the constant application of cold, wet cloths very frequently changed. When the external heat is considerable and uniform over the whole surface, the wet-sheet-pack, for an hour or more, should be employed daily, Otherwise the surface, wherever preternaturally hot, should be sponged frequently with tepid water. The bowels must be freely moved, unless diarrhœa attends, in which case fomentations should be applied to the abdomen for fifteen or twenty minutes, to be followed by the wet girdle. Water may be drank at pleasure; but no food should be allowed until the violence of the fever has materially abated.

ERYTHEMA.—This term is often confounded with Erysipelas; but is more frequently applied to local affections of an erysipelatous character. Dermatologists describe many varieties of Erythema, as *Chilblain, Carbuncle, Intertrigo*, Chafing, Burn, Mercurial, etc., which are treated of under their respective names.   6*

ESCHAR.—The crust or disorganized portion arising from the death or mortification of a part. The adjacent living tissue removes it by excreting pus between itself and the dead matter, causing the latter to fall or slough off.

ESOTERIC.—Interior, Private, in contradistinction to *Exoteric.* Esoteric causes of disease exist within the organism, as poisons introduced, or effete matter retained. Exoteric causes exist without, as malaria, heat, cold, etc.

ESOTERISM, MEDICAL.—M. SIMON has applied this term to "the *esotery,* or mystery and secrecy with which the practitioner performs his daily duties, and which, he conceives, he is compelled to adopt, by the prejudices and ignorance of his patients."

Alas! that medical men should conceive it a duty to act in a perpetual mystification, because their patients are ignorant! I fear this practice will never cure them of their ignorance and prejudices. How much better it would be to enlighten them! After all I suspect, however, this Esoterism is intended more for the benefit of the profession than the people.

ESTIVAL.—Happening in summer. Summer diseases, so called, are diarrhœa, dysentery, and cholera infantum.

ETHERIZATION.—The aggregate phenomena occasioned by the inhalation of ether. Small doses induce excitement, with more or less of mental exhilaration; large doses induce great muscular relaxation with insensibility. For the treatment see Asphyxia.

ETIOLATION.—Blanching, Paleness, whether the result of chronic disease, or from the absence of light. Bright light and abundant sunshine are among our best remedial appliances for many forms of scrofulous, anemic, and other cachectic conditions.

EUTROPHIC.—Professor DUNGLISON has introduced this term into his Medical Dictionary, for "an agent whose action is exerted on the system of nutrition, without necessarily occasioning manifest increase of any of the secretions." And he informs us that the chief Eutrophics are "*mercurials,* the preparations of *iodine, bromine, cod-liver oil,* the preparations of *gold, and silver, sulphur, sugar* and sarsaparilla." Was ever a medical muddle so bemuddled? Mercury and sugar belong to the same class of medicines. If either of Dr. DUNGLISON's Eutrophics "exert any action" on the system of nutrition, except that which is damaging and disease-producing, the fact has never yet been recorded in any medical text-book.

EVERSIO PALPEBRÆ.—Ectropion.

EXACERBATION.—An increase, or aggravation of symptoms. Often incorrectly employed as synonymous with paroxysm.

EXÆMIA, EXÆMOS.—Anæmia, Exanguous.

EXANGIA.—A term including Aneurism, and Varix.

EXANTHEM.—Exanthema. Under this term some authors comprehend all kinds of cutaneous eruptions, while others apply it only to the eruptive fevers.

EXANTHEMATICA.—Eruptive fevers.

EXANTHEMATOPHTHALMIA.—Inflammation of the eye in the course of, or succeeding, a cutaneous eruption. For treatment see Opthalmia.

EXANTHESIS.—See Efflorescence.

EXCITATION.—Excitement and stimulation are generally employed as synonymous terms. There is not so great a delusion in the world as that which mistakes excitation for augmented vitality, and stimulation for strength. The employment of stimulants is predicated on this fallacy, and alcoholic medication, which is the parent source of intemperance in the land, would have no basis, were this error corrected. For a full discussion of this subject the reader is referred to my recent work, "The True Temperance Platform."

EXCORIATION.—The abrasion of the skin from a slight wound, or an acrid excretion. Excoriated surfaces should be protected from the contact of atmospheric air, by a covering of fine flour or simple cerate.

EXCREMENT.—The waste matter and debris of the tissues— feces, urine, bile, sweat, and carbonic acid gas. The retention of effete matters is a prolific source of disease. And the accumulation of excrementitious matter in privies, stables, hog-pens, and cow-yards, is no doubt the chief cause of contagious diseases. If people would be cleanly, within and without, many of the most fatal acute diseases, and a long catalogue of chronic maladies would soon disappear.

EXCRESCENCE.—A tumor which forms at the surface of organs, and especially on the skin, mucous membrane, or ulcerated surfaces, as *Warts, Hemorrhoids, Polypi, Condylomata*, etc. Some of them can be destroyed by freezing, and all are removable with caustic.

EXCRETION.—The separation and ejection of waste or excrementitious matter. The excretory organs are the skin, lungs, liver, bowels, and kidneys. Any defect in their eliminating function becomes a source of bodily impurity, and a cause of disease. Nearly all medical authors confound *excretion* and *secretion.* But they are very different processes. See Secretion.

EXFOLIATION.—The separation of the dead portions of a bone, tendon, cartilage, or aponeurosis, under the form of lamellæ or small scales. It is analogous to *sloughing* of the softer tissues. A large portion of dead and detached bone is called, *Sequestrum.*

EXHAUSTION.–Debility. Loss of strength. One of the most prolific sources of vital exhaustion, early decline, complicated disease and premature death, is the use of stimulants, which we are mistaught by the medical profession, to regard as capable of *imparting* strength, *supporting* vitality, etc.

EXHILARATION.—Intense and pleasureable mental emotion. In pathology it is a preternatural activity of the circulation with increased sensibility. The nervine medicines induce it, as tea, coffee, musk, castor, assafetida, skunk cabbage, sulphuric ether, valerian, etc. Many agents which are regarded by medical authors as possessing a combination of nervine, narcotic and stimulant properties, as alcohol, tobacco, opium, camphor, lobelia, actea, etc.,—and even the virus of the rattlesnake when taken into the stomach—will occasion, after one has become accustomed to them, and in moderate or customary doses, a high degree of exhilaration. This fact, however, does not prove their usefulness, but the contrary.

EXOMPHALUS.—Umbilical hernia. It occurs most frequently in infants. It may be easily reduced, and retained by an elastic bandage, made in the form of a girdle, with a pad in the middle, to be applied against the navel, until a cure is effected.

EXOPHTHALMIA.—Protrusion of the eye from its orbit, in consequence of an abscess or tumor in the areolar tissue. After subduing the inflammation, the treatment is entirely surgical.

EXORMIA.—See Papula.

EXOSTOSIS.—An osseous tumor. This disease may be occasioned by the rachitic, scrofulous, or gouty diathesis, caused by syphilis, or induced by mineral drugs. But it is due more to mercurial medicines administered for the cure of venereal diseases, than to all other causes combined. The whole remedial plan is expressed by the word, purification.

EXOTERIC.—See Esoteric.

EXPECTORATION.—The expulsion of mucus, pus, or other matter from the air passages. It is a symptom in pneumonia, influenza, and consumption, and often of a "common cold." Certain medicinal drugs, called expectorants, as tartar emetic, lobelia, squills, elecampagne, Senega snake root, ipecac, and many other agents which are very nauseous to the stomach, will aggravate expectoration when it exists, and thus often occasion it when it did not previously exist. They are an exceedingly pernicious class of *remedies*.

EXSANGUINITY.—See Anæmia.

EXSARCOMA.—Sarcoma.

EXSPUITION.—Spitting. This is really a disease, for persons in a strictly normal state never spit.

EXTRAVASATION.—Escape of blood or other fluids from their proper vessels into the surrounding textures. Cold applications are useful to promote absorption.

FAINTING.—Faintness, Fainting Fit. See Syncope.

FALLING OF THE BOWELS.—See Proctocele.

FALLING OF THE WOMB.—See Prolapsus Uteri.

FALSE CONCEPTION.—See Mole.

FALSE MEMBRANE.—The adventitious formation on mucous surfaces, in cases of croup, diptheria etc.

FALSE PLEURISY.—Stitch in the side, Pleuralgia, Pleurodynia.

FALSE PERIPNEUMONY.—Bastard Pleurisy. Pseudo-Pneumonia. A term applied to cases of Pneumonia, in which the attending fever has the nervous form of typhus—properly, "*Nervous Typhoid Pneumonitis.*" The modern "cattle disease," "*Pleura-Pneumonia*" is this form of inflammation of the lungs.

FAMILY DISEASES.—See Hereditary.

FANCY MARK.—Nævus.

FANTOM.—Phantom. In pathology the term applies to disorderly mental recognitions of objects—the spectres and images, which disturb the patient, whether awake or asleep.

FARCY GLANDERS.—See Equinia.

FASTIDIUM.—Squeamishness. Easily affected with nausea.

FAT.—In a pathological sense the term means corpulence, or obesity, in which effete matters are retained in the form of fat. A fattening process is, therefore, a disease-producing process, let the lovers of fat meats, and the admirers of fat persons say what they will. With some semi-civilized and savage nations corpulency is regarded as the highest possible personal accomplishment. Captain SPEKE in his late African explorations to discover the source of the Nile, made the acquaintance of African princes and kings, whose wives were so fattened that they were unable to stand erect, but obliged to "go on all fours," and the children of the colored nobility were compelled to suck milk several hours a day to promote the desired plumpness. A fattened hog is now on exhibition in this city whose combined weight of grease and scrofula, is said to be fourteen hundred pounds, with a fair prospect of accumulating to a ton. In the days of the New York Crystal Palace, we saw a swinish monstrosity on exhibition, which was said to weigh seventeen hundred pounds. The animal was unable even to *stand* on all fours.

The celebrated showman, Professor Barnum, of the American Museum, of this city, often has "the most extraordinary sights in the world," in the shape of adipose humanity. But enough on this theme. The remedy is, plainer food and less of it.

Fatty Degeneration.—This term is applied to a morbid process, by which the glandular structures are rendered soft and oleaginous. The liver is most subject to this condition. The cause is, too much of those articles which the chemico-physiologists term "calorifacient," or "respiratory" food. Geese and other poultry are confined in a dark, warm room, stuffed with carbonaceous food, by means of which their livers swell up to a large size, and acquire the condition of "fatty degeneration," and make a dainty delicacy for the depraved taste of the carnivorous epicure. Exercise, and "low fare," are the remedies for degenerate livers, whether in man or animals.

Fatuitas.—Mental Imbecility, Dementia, Idiocy.

Favosus.—A state of ulceration, resembling honeycomb.

Favus.—Porrigo.

Febricula.—A slight Fever, Ephemera.

Febris.—Fever, which see.

Feigned Diseases.—Many are the simulated, or pretended diseases by means of which impostors have undertaken to obtain favors, escape punishment, and military duty, and astonish their fellow beings. A complete catalogue would occupy too much of my space. Suffice it to say that spasmodic diseases, as catalepsy, chorea, convulsions, and epilepsy are most easily simulated. Local inflammations are readily excited by means of irritant drugs. Fevers are produced by stimulants; cachexias are made manifest by hard-drinking and going without sleep. Bowel complaints are readily manufactured with purgative medicines, or any of the cure-all pills in market. Cutaneous affections are easily made to appear by means of acids and irritants, antimonial ointment, for example, etc., etc. The examining physician is sometimes obliged to tax his ingenuity to the utmost, in order to detect them.

FEVER.—A simultaneous and prominent disturbance of all the bodily functions, attended with paroxysms of cold, hot, and sweating stages. *Fever* and *disease* may almost be regarded as synonymous, for there is scarcely a symptom of any disease, aside from structural lesions, which may not be present in some form or stage of fever. When, therefore, we know how to treat fever, in all its stages, and complications, we have very nearly mastered the Healing Art. And the rule is exceedingly simple. It is to regulate, balance, or direct the remedial action—very different indeed from the practice of the drug system, which mainly consists in suppressing the remedial effort, and counteracting the symptoms. Fevers are seldom intrinsically dangerous, though multitudes die of them every year.

The divisions and varieties of fever recognized by medical authors are multitudinous. The only important distinctions, however, for all practical purposes, are into *Inflammatory*, *Putrid*, and *Nervous*, which terms correspond with the *entonic*, *typhus*, and *typhoid* of medical books and journals. *Simple* fevers are those which are not, in their early stages, complicated with any considerable local affection. Small-pox, measles, scarlatina, erysipelas, miliaria, and plague, are called *eruptive* fevers or *exanthems*. Fevers are also denominated *idiopathic* or *primary*; but when the fever is preceded by a local disease, as consumption, it is said to be *symptomatic* or *secondary*, as *hectic*. Very dangerous fevers are termed *malignant*, and mild ones *non-malignant*. Many cases of mild fevers are rendered malignant by mal-medication. Lastly, fevers are entonic or atonic, high or low, dynamic or adynamic, sthenic or asthenic, or inflammatory or typhoid in *diathesis*, and ephemeral, continued, remittent or intermittent in *type*.

The Hygienic treatment of all forms of fever is exceedingly simple, and is all resolvable into good nursing. Few patients would ever die of fever, if the whole treatment was left to the uneducated instincts and common sense of the people.

When the circulation and temperature are unequal, cold wet cloths are to be applied to the parts which are preternaturally hot, and warm applications made to the parts which are preternaturally cold. Usually, in these cases, the head is hot and the feet and lower extremities cold. When the body is disposed to much chilliness, warm blankets, or bottles of hot water should be applied to the sides and armpits. When the whole surface is moderately hot, tepid or cool ablutions should be employed frequently, and if the heat be very great, the wet-sheet pack is preferable. Griping or neuralgic pain is to be quieted with fomentations, and pain accompanied with heat and tension may be relieved with cold applications. It is always desirable to move the bowels freely with tepid water enemas at the outset, unless there is tendency to diarrhœa, in which case small enemas of cold water should be administered. The patient may drink pure water *ad libitum*, and may be allowed the moderate use of ripe, juicy fruits. No food, save thin gruel and a moderate allowance of fruit, should be permitted, until the crisis of the disease, or until the violence of the paroxysms, has materially abated. Free ventilation is always important; while all sources of irritation or annoyance should be carefully avoided. The patient should be kept as quiet as possible, and at all times be allowed to sleep as much as he can. Lights should not be allowed in the room, except when waiting on the patient, nor should whispering night-watchers be tolerated for a moment. After the crisis has occurred no very cold bath, nor the pack, should be employed, whatever the degree of feverishness, or however violent may be the "relapse." Tepid ablutions, warm or cold local applications are all the bathing processes required in any form, state or stage of fever, *after* the crisis or "turn of the fever" has taken place. Mischief has been done by incompetent practitioners from not knowing or not observing this rule.

The only really dangerous features of fevers are the *complications*. These are mainly, *hemorrhage, tympanitis, diarrhœa, vomiting, retention or suppression of urine, compression of the brain, determination of blood, local inflammations and congestions, profuse sweating*, and *involuntary evacuations;* but all these affections, when occurring as the incidents of fevers, require precisely the same treatment as when occurring as idiopathic affections. The reader is referred to these terms for special instruction.

FEVER, ADENO-MENINGEAL.—Various forms of fever, when attended with considerable mucus excretion, especially from the alimentary canal, have received this appellation. They have also been called Pituitous Fever, Mucus Fever, Mesenteric Fever, Catarrhal Fever, Gastro-Bronchitis, etc.

FEVER AND AGUE.—See Fever, Intermittent.

NOSOLOGICAL ARRANGEMENT OF THE SIMPLE FEVERS.

Cont'd Fevers

1. EPHEMERAL—One day Fever.
2. INFLAMMATORY—Synochus—General Inflammation.
3. TYPHOID. { Yellow Fever, Nervous Fever, Putrid Fever. } { Ship Fever, Spotted Fever, Camp Fever, Jail Fever, Hospital Fever. }
4. REMITTENT. { Nervous Remittent, Putrid Remittent, } Marsh Fever.
5. INTERMITTENT. { Quotidian—Everyday Ague, Tertian—Third day Ague, Quartan—Fourth day Ague. }
6. SYMPTOMATIC. { Hectic Fever, Puerperal Fever, Mesenteric Fever, Milk Fever. }
7. ERUPTIVE. { Small Pox, Chicken-Pox, Cow-Pox, Measles, Scarlatina, Erysipelas, Miliria, Plague. }

FEVER, ADYNAMIC.—Adynamic is employed in the sense of atonic, feeble, prostration of the vital powers, etc., and is applied to low fevers, particularly to the various forms of typhus or typhoid fevers.

FEVER, AFRICAN.—A fever which prevails on the Western coast of Africa. It is regarded by medical authors as a "malignant, bilious remittent," and is really a severe remittent of the *putrid* form.

FEVER, ALGID.—A term applied to a very pernicious and fatal form of intermittent, accompanied by extreme coldness.

FEVER, ANOMALOUS.—A fever whose course and type are irregular has been so called.

FEVER, APHONIC.—A form of intermittent in which the voice is lost during the paroxysm.

FEVER, APOPLECTIC.—Any fever attended with apoplectic symptoms.

FEVER, ARTICULAR ERUPTIVE.—This term is applied to Dengue; also to Articular Rheumatism.

FEVER, ARTIFICIAL.—Fever induced by Stimulants.

FEVER, ASTHENIC.—Low fever.   The term is usually applied to typhus.

FEVER, ASTHMATIC.—A pernicious intermittent accompanied with Asthmatic difficulty of breathing.   The asthmatic symptom is atributable to great congestion or enlargement of the liver.

FEVER, ATAXO-ADYNAMIC.—Fever characterized by nervousness and great debility.   The term has been applied to the nervous form of typhus.

FEVER, BARCELONA.—A form of Yellow Fever which has prevailed in Barcelona, sometimes called *Bastard* or *Illegitimate* Fever.

FEVER, BILIOUS.—The term *bilious*. is frequently applied to the common remittent fever of autumn. It is also sometimes applied to a mild form of putrid continued fever—the *synochus* of the nosologists.   The term *bilious remittent*, has been applied to yellow fever, though this is really of the continued type.

FEVER, BOA VISTA.—A form of Yellow Fever which was very fatal at Fernando Po, in 1845, termed also "*malignant bilious remittent*.

FEVER, BONA.—A malignant form of Remittent or Marsh Fever, which prevailed among the troops of the garrison of Bona, in Algeria, from 1832 to 1835.

FEVER, BORN.—See Dengue.

FEVER, CAMP.—Putrid Typhus.

FEVER, CARDIALGIC.—A severe Intermittent accompanied with violent pain in the stomach during the paroxysm.

FEVER, CARDITIC.—Intermittent fever accompanied with violent pain in the region of the heart.

FEVER, CATARRHAL.—See Fever, Adeno-Meningeal.

FEVER, CEPHALALGIC.—Intermittent fever with intense pain in the head.

FEVER, CEPHALIC.—The feverish disturbance which accompanies hydrocephalus.

FEVER, CEREBRAL.—Brain Fever. See Inflammation of the Brain.

FEVER, CHILDBED.—Peritonitis. Puerperal Fever. Acute inflammation of the peritoneum, or lining membrane of the abdomen, with low or typhoid fever. Lying-in women are the subjects of it. It is attended with heat and tension of the abdomen, with frequent pulse, thirst, coated tongue, and all the indications of fever of the atonic diathesis. There is usually obstinate constipation, but in some cases diarrhœa exists. Medical authors recommend diametrically opposite methods of treatment; some advising copious bleeding, salts, antimony, and other antiphlogistic agents, while others insist on opium and other stimulants as the proper remedies. As might be expected, *apriori*, the result of both plans of medication is fearfully fatal, the deaths averaging more than seventy-five per cent. We have never found any difficulty in promptly curing the disease with Hygienic appliances. The preternatural heat and tenderness of the abdomen can be relieved in a few hours, by the repeated application of cold wet cloths, care being taken to keep the feet and extremities warm; after which the bowels are to be moved with enemas of tepid or moderately warm water; the whole surface should be sponged with water just pleasantly cool, two or three times in each twenty-four hours, until the fever is permanently roduced. In all other respects the patient should be managed according to the general rules which apply to the treatment of all fevers. When the lochial discharge has been suddenly suppressed, there will be "rush of blood to the head" with intense headache, or delirium, in which case, cold applications should be made to the head, warm to the feet, with warm hip-baths, or, if the patient is not able to sit up, fomentations may be applied to the abdomen.

FEVER, CHOLERIC.—Intermittent Fever, with biliary derangement resembling Cholera Morbus.

FEVER, CHOLERIC, OF INFANTS.—Cholera Infantum.

FEVER, CHRONIC.—Symptomatic Fever. Hectic Fever.

FEVER, COLLIQUATIVE.—Various forms of fever attended with profuse discharges and rapid emaciation, have received this appellation.

FEVER, COMATOSE.—See Fever Apoplectic.

FEVER, CONGESTIVE.—The term, congestive, is employed quite as loosely in medical nomenclature as is the term bilious. In both cases, a word, which only expresses a symptom is made to designate the disease. This word, congestive, is applied promiscuously to all fevers, whether intermittent, remittent, or continued, in which there is disproportionate accumulation of blood or obstruction in any organ so that the hot stage of the paroxysm—"reaction" as the books have it, is imperfectly or not at all developed. In this form of fever many patients die in the cold stage, and within a few hours after the "attack," as it is absurdly called. Warm applications, general and local fomentations, the hot or tepid bath, warm wet-sheet pack, etc., are the proper remedial appliances, until the hot stage is fully developed, after which the disease is to be treated on "general principles."

FEVER, CONSECUTIVE.—The feverishness which follows the sudden suppression of evacuations by narcotics and stimulants, as when the alvine dejections are arrested by means of large doses of opium, morphine, or brandy. If the cholera is "cured" this way, a bad matter is only made worse, as the patient is certain to die of the "Consecutive Fever."

FEVER, CONTINENT.—This term is usually applied to Synochus or *Inflammatory Fever;* but is not unfrequently employed to designate any mild form of fever of the continued type. The *continued type* of fever may be known by two excerbations of the hot stage daily, one in the morning, and a more considerable one in the afternoon or evening. The continued fevers are, the *Inflammatory* or *entonic,* the various forms of typhus or typhoid, as *Yellow, Spotted, Camp, Ship, Jail, Hospital, Sweating, Sinking,* etc., and the eruptive fevers—*Small-pox, Measles, Scarlatina, Erysipelas, Miliaria* and *Plague.* Visceral inflammations are accompanied with fever of the continued type.

FEVER, CONVULSIVE.—Intermittent or Remittent Fever accompanied with Spasmodic Symptoms.

FEVER, DELIRIOUS.—Intermittent Fever with delirium.

FEVER, DEPURATORY.—A term applied to fevers which were supposed to have the property of purifying the blood, or in which such an effect was produced. All fevers have this tendency. Indeed, the very essence of fever is, a process of purification, and happy would it be for the sufferers if their physicians could practically recognize this truth.

FEVER, DIAPHORETIC.—Intermittent Fever with excessive sweating.

FEVER, DIARY.—Ephemeral or One Day Fever.

FEVER, DIGESTIVE.—Prof. DUNGLISON says, "the chilliness, followed by increased heat and quickness of pulse, which frequently accompanies digestion." Indigestive Fever would be a better term, as these symptoms do not exist when digestion is well performed. The sole cause of this fever is food of improper quality or quantity, or extraneous matters taken with the food.

FEVER, DOUBLE.—An Intermittent which has two paroxysms in a given time, instead of one.

FEVER, DOUBLE-QUARTAN.—A fever whose paroxysms occur two days in succession, and fail on the third day.

FEVER, DOUBLE-QUOTIDIAN.—An Intermittent whose paroxysms return twice every day at corresponding hours.

FEVER, DOUBLE-TERTIAN.—An Intermittent whose paroxysms return every day.

FEVER, DYNAMIC.—Synocha.   Remittent fever.

FEVER, EPILEPTIC.—Intermittent accompanied with Epilepsy.

FEVER, EROTIC.—Fever occasioned by unrequited love.

FEVER, ERRATIC.—Dengue.   Hectic.

FEVER, FAINTING.—A singular and fatal epidemic, resembling cholera, which prevailed at Teheran, Persia, in 1842.

FEVER, GANGRENOUS.—Fever accompanied with gangrene of various parts, especially of the limbs and genital organs.

FEVER, GASTRALGIC.—Intermittent with burning pain in the epigastrium.

FEVER, GASTRIC.—A term sometimes applied to what is commonly called Bilious Fever.

FEVER, GASTRO-ADYNAMIC.—This term has been applied to those forms of typhoid fever in which there is much gastric or biliary derangement.

FEVER, GASTRO-ANGIOTENIC.—"A fever," says DUNGLISON, "in which the symptoms of bilious are united to those of inflammatory fever."   In plainer English, this means, a mild form of *Putrid Typhus*.

FEVER, GASTRO-ATAXIC.—This absurd phrase is applied to Putrid Typhus, when the diathesis is a little lower, or the debility a little greater, than in the preceding case.

FEVER, GIBRALTER.—Yellow Fever.

FEVER, HÆMOPTOIC.—Intermittent attended with periodical hemorrhage from the lungs.

FEVER, HAY.—A periodical Catarrhal affection, with general feverishness, which affects some persons in the Summer

Season. It has also been called Hay Asthma, Summer Catarrh, Rose Catarrh, and Summer Bronchitis.

FEVER, HEBDOMADAL. — A fever whose paroxysms return weekly, and on the same day. It is no doubt purely imaginary.

FEVER, HECTIC.—Secondary, or Symptomatic Fever. It is a form of remittent which attends the later stages of chronic diseases, when great emaciation or some degree of disorganization has taken place. It can only be cured by removing the primary malady. A tepid ablution with the hot-and-cold foot-bath, and, perhaps, cool wet cloths to the head, are applicable to the fever part of the malady.

FEVER, HEPATIC. — Intermittent with violent pain in the region of the liver.

FEVER, HILL.—A form of remittent which has prevailed in the hilly districts of India.

FEVER, HOSPITAL.—A form of Putrid Typhus.

FEVER, HUMORAL.—A term applied to fever in which deterioration of the humours is suspected. It will apply equally to any and every form of fever, only differing in degree.

FEVER, HUNGARY.—An epidemic typhus which has prevailed among the soldiers in barracks, in Hungary.

FEVER, HYDROPHOBIC.—"Pernicious Intermittent with dread of liquids," says DUNGLISON.

FEVER, HYSTERIC. — Intermittent with Hysterical paroxysms.

FEVER, ICTERIC.—Fever accompanied with Jaundice.

FEVER, INFANTILE REMITTENT. — Worm-Fever; Irritative Fever. A fever occurring in childhood, and caused by indigestible food or constipated bowels.

FEVER, INFLAMMATORY.—Synocha; Cauma.

The Entonic Diathesis.—Inflammatory Fever is the least dangerous of all forms of fever, and, although a multitude of deaths occur annually, I have no shadow of doubt they are attributable to the medication, and not to the malady. I have never known nor heard of a person dying of this disease under Hygienic treatment. The disease may be known by *strong pulse*, white tongue with red eyes, uniform heat, and dryness of the skin, turgescence and florid redness of the whole surface, with a diminution of all the excretions. The mental functions are never very much disturbed.

The treatment is very simple, and should be always successful. The bowels should be moved freely with enemas of tepid water at first, and subsequently, whenever there is hardness, tension and uneasiness in the abdomen. The patient may drink pure water of any temperature most agreeable, and in any quantity he is inclined to. The whole surface should be sponged with cool or cold water as either may be most pleasant, as often as the heat rises much above the normal standard; or, if practicable, the wet-sheet pack may be employed once or twice each day. When the superficial heat is very great, double wet sheets should be used. The prolonged tepid full bath is well adapted to this form of fever, though it is not so agreeable to the patient as the wet-sheet pack. No food should be taken until the skin becomes moist and the coat of the tongue begins to disappear.

FEVER, INSIDIOUS.—A term applied to fevers which do not seem dangerous at first, but subsequently become malignant. I suspect these superventions of malignancy are more frequently due to maltreatment than to any other cause. The late Prince ALBERT, Senator DOUGLASS, Count CAVOUR, General SUMNER, THOMAS STARR KING, and many other distinguished names I could mention, are illustrations.

FEVER, INTERMITTENT.—This type of fever—ague and fever —is characterized by a complete subsidence of the hot stage of the paroxysm, constituting what is called an *intermission*, during which the patient is often enabled to attend to ordinary duties or labors. The paroxysms may occur daily, or every second or third day, or even twice a day.

Warm foot-baths, fomentations to the abdomen, bottles of hot water etc., to the sides and arm-pits are applicable to the cold stage. When the whole surface becomes preternaturally hot, tepid ablutions, or the wet-sheet pack, according to the degree of heat, are to be employed. During the period of intermission the patient should avoid fatigue, and be extremely careful and abstemious in the dietary.

FEVER, JAIL.—Putrid Typhus.

FEVER, LOCHIAL.—A feverish disturbance which frequently occurs during the discharge of the lochia.

FEVER, LUNG.—Inflammation of the Lungs. Pneumonia, Pneumonitis; sometimes applied to Influenza.

FEVER, MALIGNANT.—Any fever which is dangerous may be said to be malignant. Plague and spotted fever, are always malignant. Various forms of typhoid and eruptive fevers may be either malignant or non-malignant.

FEVER, MALIGNANT PESTILENTIAL.—A phrase which has been applied to severe forms of Remittent, and sometimes to Yellow Fever.

FEVER, MASKED.—Dumb Ague, Dead Ague. Terms applied to disguised or irregular forms of intermittent.

FEVER, MENINGO-GASTRIC.—Stomach Fever. The feverishness of indigestion.

FEVER, MESENTERIC.—A term employed by BAGLIVI, and applied to fevers which other authors designate as Bilious, Mucous, Synochus, etc.

FEVER, MILIARY.—Millet-Seed Rash. See Miliary Fever.

FEVER, MILK.—The febrile disturbance which precedes or accompanies the secretion of milk in women recently delivered. Tepid or cool wet cloths to the breasts, frequently changed, and warm foot-baths are the specialities of treatment. Constipation must be removed or obviated, and the general feverishness removed at once, by means of the full warm bath and tepid ablutions, or a lingering illness with a "broken breast" may be the result.

FEVER, MIXED.—Synochus; Putrid Typhus.

FEVER, NEPHRITIC.—Intermittent fever with pain in the region of the kidneys during the paroxysm.

FEVER, NERVOUS.—Typhus Mitior of CULLEN; Entonic fever of some modern authors. This is the *Typhoid Fever* of those authors who make a distinction between *Typhus* and *Typhoid*—a distinction, however, without a difference.

Nervous fever, of whatever type, always requires gentle treatment. No violent shocks or very cold baths can be tolerated, or should be prescribed. Careful nursing is here the best medication in an emphatic sense. Tepid ablutions, cool or cold applications to the head, warm applications to the extremities, cold compresses or hot fomentations, as either may be indicated at any time, as best calculated to balance the circulation, are the essentials of the remedial plan. Quiet and rest are of especial importance in this form of fever. The very young, very old, and very feeble, are peculiarly the subjects of it.

FEVER, NIGER.—A malignant Remittent Fever, which proved fatal to many in the expeditions sent out by the British government to explore the Niger, in 1841-2, has been so designated.

FEVER, NONANE.—"A suppositious fever, whose paroxysms recur every ninth day, or every eighth day."

FEVER, OCTANE.—An intermittent whose paroxysms recur every eighth day.

FEVER, PALUDAL.—Marsh or Remittent Fever, Elodes.

FEVER, PERIODICAL.—Intermittent or Remittent Fever.

FEVER, PERNITIOUS.—This term has been applied to severe or malignant intermittent.

FEVER, PESTILENTIAL OF CATTLE.—Murr. Murrain. A disease having a close resemblance to small-pox which affects cattle.

FEVER, PLEURITIC.—Intermittent or Remittent Fever accompanied with inflammation of the pleura. Pleuralgia, or "stitch in the side" is often mistaken for pleurisy.

FEVER, PNEUMONIC.—Pneumonia. Inflammation of the lungs. Intermittent with symptoms of inflammation of the lungs has been termed, though very absurdly, Pulmonic Fever.

FEVER, PSEUDO.—Feverishness. General Irritation.

FEVER, PUERPERAL.—Peritonitis. See Childbed Fever.

FEVER, PUKING.—Milk Sickness.

FEVER, PURULENT.—Fever which accompanies suppuration.

FEVER, PUTRID.—This is the most common form of fever, always was, and always will be. Fever being essentially a process of purification, its *causes* are necessarily impurities in the system, whether in the form of retained effete matters, or poisons. These occasion grossness, or putrescency of the blood, with its consequences—morbid secretions and foul excretions. The term, *putrid*, applies properly to those forms of fever in which grossness, foulness, or impurity of the whole mass of blood, is the obvious and most prominent condition. The milder forms of putrid fever, are often termed *Bilious, Synochus*, "Bilious Fever with Typhoid symptoms," "Bilious running into Typhoid," etc. The severer forms—those dependent on extreme grossness—are the malignant forms of Typhus or Typhoid, as *Spotted, Ship, Jail, Camp, Hospital, Yellow, Sinking*, etc., fevers. Many of the visceral inflammations, as *Diptheria, Pneumonia*, and *Dysentery*, are frequently accompanied with putrid fever, have been denominated *malignant* or *typhoid*. The eruptive fevers—*Small-pox, Measles*, and *Scarlatina*, are sometimes *putrid*, and are then termed *typhoid* or *malignant*. Erysipelas and miliaria are always putrid, though sometimes moderately so, while the plague is always extremely putrid—the worst and most malignant form of Putrid Typhus known. Putrid Fever, in all its forms, varieties and complications, is easily recognized by a few characteristic and prominent symptoms—the crimson or dark flush, the dark-red, dirty-yellow, or black tongue, velvety redness of the eyes, foul breath, fetid excretions, spotted, mottled, or blotched appearance of the skin, delirium, etc. Hemorrhages, congestions, abscesses, carbuncles, etc., are more liable to occur in this form of fever, than in the nervous or inflammatory forms.

The treatment, as in all other forms of fever, must be regulated by the circulation and temperature of the patient.

The more feeble the pulse, the warmer should the baths be. Warm, tepid, cool or cold ablutions may be best in different cases. In the mild cases, when the whole surface is preternaturally hot, the plan of treatment does not vary much from that applicable to inflammatory fever. As there is a constant tendency to congestion of, or determination to, the brain, lungs, or liver, indicated by delirium, or coma, difficult respiration, or prolonged chills, with extreme yellowness of the eyes and surface, great care must be taken to maintain the balance of circulation, as in cases of nervous fever. When the local heat and pain are considerable, cold applications must be constantly applied, and when there is tendency to ulceration, as in diptheria, malignant scarlet fever, and putrid sore throat, ice should be freely employed. Hemorrhagic tendencies require cool applications locally, warm to the extremities, bits of ice or sips of ice-water frequently taken into the stomach. The utmost attention should be given to ventilation, frequent changes of bedding and linen, and the instant removal of all effete or excrementitious matters.

FEVER, QUINTAN.—A fever whose paroxysms are supposed to return every fifth day. Doubtful.

FEVER, QUOTIDIAN.—Red Tongue. The term has been applied to Typhus.

FEVER, RED TONGUE.—A form of Typhus which has prevailed in Kentucky.

FEVER, REGULAR.—Intermittent; whose paroxysms have a determinate order and succession of stages.

FEVER, RELAPSING.—This term has been lately applied to the *secondary* fever which occurs after the patient has had ordinary, simple fever, passed the crisis, a critical period, and been apparently convalescent for one, two, three, or more days. It is nothing more nor less than a *drug disease*, occasioned by the medicines which have been administered to cure the original fever. It is attended with profuse sweating, and never occurs in patients who are treated Hygienically. The rationale of Relapsing Fever is easily explained. After the primary fever has "run its course," and the body has rested long enough to recover a good degree of its normal sensibilities and vigor, it makes an effort to expel the drugs which have been accumulating under the dosings of the doctors; and this effort is all there is of this form of fever. The only treatment required is perfect rest, tepid sponge baths occasionally, and strict attention to all hygienic conditions.

FEVER, REMITTENT.—Marsh Fever, Autumnal Fever. The Remittent *type* of fever differs from the Intermittent in this: There is a *partial*, instead of a *complete*, subsidence of the hot stage of the paroxysm. Remittent Fever has one paroxysm every twenty-four hours. It may be of either the *putrid* or *nervous* form, and malignant or non-malignant. As this form of fever is intermediate between Intermittent and continued, so the treatment should be. All of the rules I have indicated as applicable to the management of putrid and nervous fevers are just as applicable here, reference being had to the intensity and duration of the hot stage of the paroxysm. The various forms of Remittent Fever are liable to the same accidents or complications as are the various forms of Putrid and Nervous fevers of the continued type, and require precisely the same treatment. The term, Bilious Remittent, is usually applied to the mild, and malignant Remittent to the severe form of the disease.

FEVER, SCORBUTIC.—Feverishness accompanying Scurvy.

FEVER, SEASONING.—See Fever, Strangers'.

FEVER, SECONDARY.—In a strict sense this term is applied to the febrile disturbance which recurs in certain febrile affections, after having once ceased, as in the Small-pox and other eruptive fevers.

FEVER, SEPTAN.—Intermittent, whose paroxysms recur every six days, and consequently on the seventh.

FEVER, SEXTAN.—A fever which recurs every five days, and consequently on the sixth.

FEVER, SHIP.—A form of Putrid Typhus.

FEVER, SIMPLE.—Any fever uncomplicated with visceral inflammation, exanthem, or local disorganization. Simple fever may be of either the continued, remittent, or intermittent type, or of either the entonic or atonic diathesis.

FEVER, SIMPLE CONTINUED.—The term is applied indiscriminately to Inflammatory, Putrid, or Nervous fever, when they are of a mild form.

FEVER, SINGULTOUS.—Fever accompanied with hiccough.

FEVER, SINKING.—Typhus Syncopalis. A malignant form of Putrid Typhus.

FEVER, SPOTTED.—Putrid Typhus, accompanied with spots or blotches on the skin, absurdly called "Cerebro-Spinal Meningitis," on the supposition that the disease consisted essentially of an inflammation of the coats of the brain and spinal marrow. The horrid conglomeration of remedies—blistering, cupping, leeching, bleeding, mercurializing, antiphlogisticating, and alcoholizing—has been as disastrous to the patients as the theory is nonsensical in medical science.

FEVER, STERCORAL.—Fever induced by accumulated fecal matters in the intestines.

FEVER, STOMACHIC.—Gastric Fever; Indigestion.

FEVER, STRANGERS'.—Acclimating or Seasoning Fever. Yellow or remittent fever to which strangers are especially liable, and which is endemic in certain places.

FEVER, SUBCONTINUAL.—Remittent.

FEVER, SUBINTRANT.—Intermittent; in which one paroxysm is scarcely finished before another begins.

FEVER, SWEATING.—Sudor Anglicus. Typhus Fever accompanied with profuse sweating.

FEVER, SYNCOPAL.—Intermittent, accompanied with one or more faintings in every paroxysm.

FEVER, SYNOCHOID.—Synochus.

FEVER, SYPHILTIC.—Feverishness accompanying Syphilis.

FEVER, TERTIAN.—Intermittent; whose paroxysm return on the third day, consequently every two days.

FEVER, TRAGIC.—Fever accompanied with delirium, during which the patient declaims like an actor.

FEVER, TRAUMATIC.—The fever which supervenes on wounds and surgical operations.

FEVER, TYPHOID OR TYPHUS.—Continued Fever of the *atonic* diathesis. The fever of the visceral inflammations, when not *entonic*, is typhoid; and the same is true of the Exanthems or Eruptive fevers. Thus we have typhoid pneumonitis, typhoid dysentery, typhoid or confluent small-pox, typhoid or black measles, typhoid or malignant scarlatina etc.

FEVER, VERMINOUS.—Worm Fever; Helminthropyra. Fever occasioned by worms in the alimentary canal.

FEVER, VERNAL.—Fever occurring in the Spring.

FEVER, VESICULAR.—Pemphigus.

FEVER, WALCHEREN.—Gall-Sickness. The remittent and intermittent, which affected British troops attached to the expedition to Walcheren, in 1809.

FEVER, WATER BRAIN.—Internal Hydrocephalus.

FEVER, YELLOW.—A form of Putrid Typhus, accompanied with yellowness of the skin, sense of burning heat in the region of the stomach, and commonly with an ejection of vitiated bile, called "*a black vomit.*" Though of the continued type, it has one peculiar feature approximating the remittent, which is, a remission on the second or third day. The treatment is in all respects the same as for putrid fever, of which it is one of its many varieties. So far as I have heard, the Hygienic treatment, in New Orleans, Mobile, Vicksburg, Nicaragua, and other places where it has been employed more or less, has been uniformly successful. Under drug treatment it is as fatal, nearly, as is Spotted Fever when treated drugopathically.

FEVERISHNESS.—A disturbance of the temperature and circulation resembling a slight fever.

FICUS.—Sycosis, Sycoma.   A fleshy excrescence on the eyelids, chin, tongue, anus, or organs of generation, hanging by a pedicle, or formed by a fig.   It may be hard or soft. They may be readily destroyed with ligature or caustic.

FIDGETS.—Restlessness.   Great fatigue, constipation, any considerable local irritation, or the use of stimulants, nervines, or narcotics, may occasion it.   The remedy consists in removing the cause.

FISSURE.—In pathology, a long, narrow, superficial ulcer, most frequently affecting the rectum or lower bowel, but sometimes the os uteri and vagina.   They are exceedingly annoying, and are attended with a burning or stinging sensation, always aggravated on the patient becoming warm in bed. Enemas of cold water, with a plain vegetable dietary, and a few touches of caustic will remove them.   Anhydrous sulphate of zinc is the best application.

FISTULA.—A sinuous ulcer, the opening or outlet of which is narrow, and the disease prolonged, by an altered texture of the parts.   A fistula is *complete* when there are two openings, and *incomplete* when there is only one.   In order to cure them it is necessary to destroy its lining membrane, which is somewhat analogous to mucous membrane, and excretes an acrid fluid.   This may be done with various caustics, of which sulphate of zinc, proto-chloride of iron, and tincture of iodine are among the best.   Those which are dependent on diseased bone, cartilage, or tendon, do not heal until after the exfoliation of the diseased part.   Fistulas of excretory ducts are produced by an injury of the duct itself, or by the retention and accumulation of the fluids to which they give passage.

FISTULA IN ANO.—This is the most common form of fistula, and generally arises from some mechanical pressure or impediment.   Hardened and accumulated feces are the most frequent cause.   Injections of a strong solution of anhydrous sulphate of zinc is the best remedy.   But this will not succeed unless the bowels are kept in good condition by a proper dietary.

FISTULOUS.—Relating to, or resembling, a fistula.
7*

FLATULENCE.—Bombus, Windy. Accumulation of gas in the alimentary canal, or its emission by the mouth or anus. It is symptomatic of indigestion, and is often the cause of severe colic. Warm water internally, and fomentations externally, are the remedies.

FLESH, PROUD.—Fungosity.

FLUCTUATION.—The motion or the undulation of a fluid collected in any cavity, which is felt by pressure or by percussion.

FLUOR.—Flux.

FLUOR ALBUS.—Whites. See Leucorrhœa.

FLUSH.—Redness occasioned by accumulation of blood in the capillaries of the face, as the *flush* or *blush* of emotion, or of hectic fever.

FLUX.—A discharge. Usually applied to dysentery.

FLUX, BILIOUS.—Cholera Morbus.

FLUX, BLOODY. -Dysentery, Catarrh, Influenza, Spermatorrhœa, Salivation, Hemorrhoids, the menstrual discharge, etc., are termed fluxes in some nosologies.

FLUXION.—Determination. An increased flow of blood or other fluid to any part.

FORMITES.—A term applied to substances which are supposed to retain contagious affluvia, as cotton and woolen goods, feathers, etc.

FORMICA.—The ant. Also the name of a black wart, *verruca formicaria*, the pain of which resembles the biting of an ant.

FORMICATION.—A pain resembling that caused by a number of ants creeping on a part.

FRAMBŒSIA.—The Yaws. A disease of Africa and the Antilles, characterized by tumors resembling raspberries, strawberries, or champignons. They ulcerate and become infectious. They indicate extreme grossness of the body, and purification is all that need be said of the treatment.

FROSTBITE.—Congelation. Frozen parts should always be thawed very gradually, to obviate consequent inflammation. Friction or rubbing should be avoided, for the reason that the angular particles of the congealed fluids will, if disturbed, break and disorganize the tissues.

FUGACIOUS.—Symptoms which rapidly appear and disappear.

FUNGOSITY.—Proud Flesh. It requires compression in moderate cases, and in severer ones, astringents or caustics. Wounds which are treated with water dressings are seldom troubled with fungus excrescences.

FUNGUS.—Fungosity, Mycosis. Warts and vegetations which arise on the skin and on denuded surfaces; also tumors which form in the substance of the textures.

FUNGUS HÆMATODES.—A bleeding Fungus. All kinds of fungoid tumors or excrescences are to be treated with caustic, due attention being paid to the general health. The more extensive and malignant the fungus the more powerful in its disorganizing effects should be the caustic selected. Nitrate of silver, nitric acid, sulphate of zinc, carbonate of potassa, chloride of sodium, etc., afford the most convenient appliances.

FURFURACEOUS.—Resembling bran. Scurfy eruptions in which the epidermis is detached in small scales; also a bran-like sediment sometimes observed in the urine.

FURIA INFERNALIS.—A small vermiform insect, common in Sweden, whose sting occasions excruciating torture.

FUROR.—Mania, Rage. Symptomatic of many morbid conditions, which will be treated of under their respective heads.

FURUNCULUS.—Boil. A small phlegmon or abscess, having its seat in the dermoid texture. It proceeds to suppuration, and breaks and discharges pus mixed with blood. The *core* consists of dead areola tissue. Cold applications in the early stages, and fomentations or poultices, after throbbing pains are felt, constitute the remedial plan.

GALACTIA.—A redundant flow of milk. A dry and abstemious dietary is the remedy.

GALACTOHÆMIA.—A condition of blood in which it contains milk.

GALEANTHROPY.—A species of melancholy in which the patient imagines himself changed into a cat.

GALL-SICKNESS.—Nausea and headache, caused by vitiated bile.

GALL-STONES.—See Calculi, Biliary.

GANGLION.—A knot. In anatomy, applied to various structures which constitute the brains and reservoirs of the organic nervous system. In pathology, a ganglion is a hard, globular tumor, in size varying from that of a pea to that of an egg, and always situated in the course of a tendon. It contains a viscid fluid enclosed in a cyst, which is sometimes loose, but in most cases communicates by a narrow footstalk with the sheath of a tendon, or the synovial capsule of a joint. They may be removed by extirpation, incision, compression, or percussion.

GANGRENE.—Incipient mortification. It is marked by a sudden diminution of feeling; livid discoloration; detachment of the cuticle, under which a turbid fluid is effused, with crepitation, owing to the disengagement of air into the areolar tissue. Gangrene is to be regarded as one of the stages of inflammation, and should be treated with tepid, cool, or cold applications, according to the temperature of the part.

GAPING.—See Yawning.

GASTRALGIA.—Cardialgia, Hartburn.

GASTRITIS.—Inflammation of the Stomach. It is known by great anxiety; heat and pain in the epigastrium, increased by pressure, and by taking anything into the stomach; vomiting; hiccough, and general fever. The inflammation may be active, adhesive, or phlegmonous, with corresponding entonic fever, or passive, erythematic, or erysipelatous, with corresponding atonic or typhoid fever. The fever part of the affection must be managed precisely as we have indicated for simple inflammatory or typhoid fever. The local affection requires the constant application of cold wet cloths, and frequent sips of cold water. Iced-water, or pieces of ice swallowed, are not objectionable. The bowels are usually constipated, and should be freely evacuated by means of enemata of tepid water.

GASTRO-ARTHRITIS.—Gout with inflammation of the stomach.

GASTROCELE.—Hernia of the stomach. Epigastrocele.

GASTRO-CEPHALITIS.—Inflammation of the stomach and head.

GASTRODYNIA.—See Cardialgia.

GASTRO-ENTERITIS.—Inflammation of the Stomach and Bowels. BROUSSAIS absurdly referred all fevers to gastro-enteritis, as their essential nature or cause.

GASTRORRHAGIA.—See Hæmatemesis.

GASTRORRHŒA.—Cœliac Flux. A term applied to a copious excretion of mucus from the lining membrane of the stomach. It is a symptom in many cases of indigestion and liver complaint.

GENYANTRITIS.—Inflammation of the Antrum of Highmore, or cavity of the cheek-bone.

GIBBOSITAS.—A symptom of Rickets, Caries, etc. See Hump.

GIDDINESS.—Vertigo. Slight congestion of the brain, or any sudden disturbance of the circulation, may induce it.

GLANDERS.—Farcy. Equinia.

GLAUCOMA.—Paropsis Glaucosis. Opacity of the vitreous humour of the eye, or of the *tunica hydloides*; which manifests itself by a greyish, or greenish spot, apparent through the pupil. It is seldom curable.

GLAUCOSIS.—Glaucoma.

GLEET.—A muco-purulent discharge from the urethra, dependent on chronic inflammation, often the result of gonorrhœa, but more commonly the effect of the drugs which are taken to cure gonorrhœa. The local treatment consists of moderately warm hip-baths, gradually reducing the temperature to tepid, then to cool, and finally to cold. The wet-girdle is a useful adjunct. The dietary should be rigidly plain and abstemious.

GLOBUS HYSTERICUS.—Nodus Hystericus. A sensation as if a ball or round body were rising from the abdomen towards the larynx, and producing a feeling of suffocation. Hysterical persons are subject to it.

GLOSSALGIA.—Pain in the Tongue.

GLOSSITIS.—Inflammation of the Tongue. It is a rare disease, except when induced by mercurial medicine.

GLOSSOCARCINOMA.—Cancer of the Tongue.

GLOSSOCELE.—Hernia of the Tongue. A swelling of the organ so that it protrudes from the mouth. It is frequently an accompaniment of mercurial salivation. The enlargement sometimes becomes chronic, and necessitates amputation of a portion of the tongue.

GLOSSOSPASMUS.—Cramp or Spasm of the Tongue.

GLUTTONY.—Habitual indulgence in over-eating. A properly restricted diet will in due time overcome the morbid craving.

GOGGLE-EYED.—Squinting, Strabismus.

GOITRE.—See Bronchocele.

GOMPHIASIS.—Soreness of the Teeth, Odontalgia. Scurvy is the most frequent cause of looseness of the adult teeth, and inflammation is the common cause of pain in them. To purify the blood is the indication in the former case; and this, with fasting, and warm or cold applications, as either may be most soothing, is the remedial plan in the latter case.

GONAGRA.—Gout in the Knees.

GONALGIA.—Pain in the Knee.

GONARTHRITIS.—Inflammation of the Knee-joint.

GONORRHŒA.—Blennorrhœa Luodes, Urethritis. Inflammation of the urethra, with mucus discharge, the result of venereal infection. It is accompanied with more or less of heat, smarting, and difficult urination. It is readily subdued by means of prolonged tepid or cool hip-baths, repeated as often as the pain and heat increase, with full warm baths or the wet-sheet pack, and a very abstemious dietary. I have never found any difficulty in curing the worst cases in a few days in this way.

GOURD-WORM.—*Distoma Hepaticum*. It has been supposed to inhabit the liver and gall-ducts.

GOUT.—Podagra. An inflammation of the joints, usually

commencing in the small joints, and more especially the joints of the great toe. The London *Lancet*, with ludicrous gravity, informs us that the disease *selects* this part in which to *explode!*

Regular gout is an inflammatory and very painful swelling of the small joints, extending more or less to the larger, attended with indigestion and general feverishness, and subsiding in a few days. The feet should be enveloped in wet cloths, covered with dry, which should be frequently renewed until the preternatural heat subsides, and the pain and swelling are abated. Meanwhile the whole body should be " packed" daily —and when the fever is considerable, twice a day—unless the patient is very weak from colchicum, digitalis, veratrina, or other depressing drugs, in which case the warm-bath followed by the tepid ablution, or dripping sheet, is to be preferred. When the joints are permanently enlarged without much inflammatory tenderness, the douche will be advantageous. It is always important to restrict the patient to a plain, abstemious, fruit and farinaceous dietary.

When the large joints are inflamed, in persons of a gouty diathesis, the disease is called *Rheumatic Gout*. When the disease has existed for some time, and dyspeptic symptoms have become prominent, the case is termed *Atonic Gout*. When the inflammation of the joints suddenly subsides, followed by great disturbance in the head, lungs and stomach, or heart, it is called *Recedent* or *Retrocedent Gout;* and when, at the usual periods for the gouty paroxysms, some one of the organs are violently disordered without the appearance of inflammation in the joints, the malady is termed *Misplaced Gout*. The symptoms of these *irregular* forms of gout are, however, to be treated precisely as when occurring from any other causes.

GRANULAR EYELIDS.—Minute tumors effecting the eyelids. They will generally disappear in a few months on the adoption of a strict Hygienic regimen. But in some cases they require the repeated application of mild caustic, as nitrate of silver, or sulphate of zinc.

GRANULAR DEGENERATION.—BRIGHT'S Disease of the Kidney. A term applied to the disorganization of the structure of the liver—the result of chronic inflammation.

GRANULATED LIVER.—Cirrhosis.

GRANULATION.—The process by which conical, flesh-like shoots are formed at the surface of suppurating wounds and ulcers. They constitute the basis of the cicatrix.

GRAVEL.—Urinary calculi. Small concretions, similar to sand or gravel, which form in the kidneys, pass along the ureters to the bladder, and are expelled through the urethra with the urine. They are commonly composed of uric acid and animal matter. The pain occasioned by the passage of these concretions can be relieved or mitigated by fomentations or the warm hip-baths, and their further formation may be prevented by purifying the whole mass of blood; and the most effective method of doing this is the negative one—cease taking impurities into the system. The patient should not drink hard water, nor use any earthy or mineral ingredient in his dietary or with his medicine, as table salt, soda, lime, chalk, etc.

GREEN-SICKNESS.—See Chlorosis.

GRIPES, WATERY.—A disease of infants, common in England, and not differing essentially from the Cholera Infantum of this country.

GRIPPE.—A vulgar name for several catarrhal diseases which have prevailed epidemically, among which is the Influenza.

GROG-BLOSSOMS.—Gutta Rosea.

GROG-ROSES.—Gutta Rosea.

GUMBOIL.—Parulis. Small abscesses which form on the gums.

GUTTA ROSEA.—Carbuncled Face, Rosy Drop, Whelk, Copper-nose, Bottle-nose. An eruption of small suppurating tubercles. The redness commonly appears first at the end of the nose, and then spreads on both sides, and sometimes extends over more or less of the face. It is commonly the effect of "hard drinking." DUNGLISON says: "Its cure must be attempted by regular regimen, and cooling means internally; weak spirituous or saturnine lotions externally." Would it not be better to stop taking the spirituous potions inside, than to try to counteract them with spirituous lotions outside?

GUTTA SERENA.—See Amaurosis.

HÆMATEMESIS.—Vomiting of Blood. Blood ejected from the stomach is dark, grumous, and frequently mixed with the contents of the stomach. The disease is preceded by a sense of weight, oppression and pain, in the epigastric region, and often accompanied with syncope. The patient must be kept very quiet; sips of cold water or bits of ice swallowed frequently; cold wet cloths covered with dry applied over the stomach and abdomen, and the extremities kept warm. If there is feverishness, the surface should be sponged with tepid water.

HÆMATOCELE.—Blood Tumor. An effusion of blood into a cavity, or into the areolar tissue. Apply cold wet cloths.

HÆMATODES FUNGUS.—Spongoid Inflammation, Pulpy or Medullary Sarcoma, Soft Cancer, Bleeding Fungus. It is a mass of cancerous tumors, in which the inflammation is accompanied with great heat and pain, and with fungus and bleeding excrescences. For the treatment, see Cancer.

HÆMATOPISIS.—Retention of the menstrual blood in the uterus.

HÆMATURIA.—Bloody Urine. Hemorrhage of the mucous membrane of the urinary passages. It may proceed from the kidneys, bladder, or urethra. Cold wet cloths, covered with dry, applied over the abdomen; sips of cold water taken frequently, and injections of a small quantity of cold water into the rectum, (or vagina, in women,) are the remedial processes.

HÆMODIA.—Tooth-edge, Odontalgia. Pain in the teeth. It is occasioned by the contact of acid or acerb substances.

HÆMOPHTHALMIA.—Blood-shot Eye. Effusion or extravasation of blood into the structures of the eye. Apply cold water or ice

HÆMOPTYSIS.—Spitting of blood; Bleeding from the Lungs. Hemorrhages from the lungs are characterized by a florid color of the blood, and its admixture with atmospheric air giving it a frothy appearance. They are preceded by more or less cough, dyspnœa, and sense of weight and heat in the chest.

Keep the patient profoundly quiet; apply cold wet cloths covered with dry over the chest; give frequent sips of cold water, or bits of ice to be swallowed; keep the extremities warm; have the room well ventilated; and if the weather is warm, the patient should be fanned; and whenever the surface is feverish bathe it with tepid water.

HÆMORRHAGIA.—Hæmorrhage; Bleeding. A discharge from blood-vessels. The *Hæmorrhagic Diathesis* is characterized by a disposition to bleed from slight injuries, and the blood being putrescent and its corpuscles broken or dissolved, as in scurvy, putrid fevers, etc., or the tissues flabby and relaxed, as in scrofula, plethora, etc. The free use of flesh meat and fermented liquors, common salt, the preparations of iron, cod-liver oil, and many other gross foods and poisonous drugs, are efficient agents in inducing the hæmorrhagic diathesis. Regular bathing, active exercise in the open air, and plain, simple, natural food, and the avoidance of all stimulating beverages, irritating condiments, and impurities and poisons of every kind, are the remedial measures for the *diathesis*. The various forms of hemorrhage are treated of under their respective heads.

HÆMORRHOIDES.—Hæmorrhois; Piles. Livid and painful tubercles or excrescences at the lower part of the rectum, attended with a discharge of mucus or blood, are the common manifestations of this affection. Constipation, and straining at stool are the ordinary causes. In some cases the tumors inflame, with tenesmus and frequent discharges of mucus mixed with blood. These cases are often mistaken for dysentery. But the absence of fever, with little or no distention, heat, or pain in the abdomen, ought to determine a correct diagnosis. In many cases the lower bowel is so relaxed as to protrude externally with every fecal evacuation, and so tender as to be returned with great difficulty.

In the treatment a carefully regulated dietary is of the first importance. When the bowels are not disposed to move without, an enema of tepid water should be employed daily; and a small quantity of cold water should be injected after each dejection, and again at bed-time. The hip-bath should be employed once or twice a day; and if there is obstruction or inaction of the liver, the wet-girdle may be advantageously worn a part of each day. When the tumors are very hard and protruberant, they may be destroyed with nitric acid, or removed with the ligature; but in nearly all cases, if the treatment is properly managed, no surgery will be required.

A soft, red, strawberry-like elevation of the mucous membrane, constituting the most common form of internal bleeding pile, has been called *Vascular Tumor* by some authors. It may be removed by the application of caustic; but I have never had any difficulty in curing it by means of Hygienic treatment alone.

HALLUCINATION.—Illusion, Waking Dream, Phantasm. DUNGLISON says, "A *morbid* error in one of the senses." Are not all errors morbid? Is there such a thing as *normal* error? It is disordered or abnormal recognition or perception of objects, involving one or but a few of the mental powers. It is the immediate result of congestion of, or determination to the brain, or some portion of it, and requires derivative treatment, as hot-and-cold foot-baths, tepid hip-baths, etc. Constipation is the most common of the remote causes.

HAMARTHRITIS.—Universal Gout; Gout in all the Joints.

HARE-LIP.—A fissure or perpendicular division of one or both lips. It requires a surgical operation.

HEAD-ACHE.—Cephalalgia, Cephalæa. Headaches are commonly symptomatic of congestion of, or determination to the brain. No cause is so general as constipated bowels. This is why females are so much more subject to this affection than males. *Sick Headache* is owing to acrid bile in the stomach. Drink warm water until relieved, whether it occasion vomiting or not.

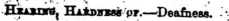

HEARING, HARDNESS OF.—Deafness.

HEART, ATROPHY OF.—A diminution in thickness of the parietes of the organ. It is rarely detected during life.

HEART, DISEASE.—Many dyspeptics with badly congested livers, and of constipated habits, are troubled with throbbing, fluttering, and irregular action of the heart, with intermittent pulse, short breath, and a multitude of distressing, but indescribable sensations, all of which are commonly disposed of by a resort to that vague phrase, *disease of the heart*. These symptoms are very frequently mistaken, even by reputable practitioners and experienced surgeons, for organic disease of the heart. But in ninety-nine cases in a hundred they are merely symptomatic of indigestion, or constipation, or both, and on restoring the general health, the heart's action will become normal.

HEART, HYPERTROPHY OF.—A thickening of the muscular substance of the organ, so that its cavities are diminished. It is seldom detected until the præcordial region becomes preternaturally prominent, and the heart's action communicates a marked jarring or vibration to the hand when placed on the cardiac region. It can only be cured or retarded by such habits of life as keep the circulation well-balanced, and the avoidance of all violent exertions, mental shocks; in short whatever disturbs the action of the heart. The dietary should always be rather abstemious.

HEART, DILATATION OF.—In this case the cavities of the organ are enlarged, with or without thickening or thinning of their parietes. The apex of the heart is lower down and more to the left than in the normal state, and the pulsations can be seen and felt over a larger space. The pulse is hard, quick, and vibratory. The shock of the heart's action is often transmitted to the whole body, and to the bed on which the patient is lying. This symptom, however, is not decisive; constipation of the bowels will induce the most violent beating of the heart, and is often mistaken for aneurism of the heart.

HEARTBURN.—Cardialgia.

Hectic Fever.—See Fever Hectic.

Helleborismus.—This term has been applied to a method of treating diseases with hellebore. It comprises the selection and preparation of the drug, the remedies for aiding it, and the precautions for obviating or lessening its pernicious effects. The philosophy of the thing is precisely like that of the modern method of treating all diseases with drugs—poisoning the system to the extent of superseding the symptoms of the original disease with those of the drug disease.

Helminthia.—See Worms.

Hemeralopia.—Nyctalopia, Day-Vision, Night Blindness, Hen Blindness. An affection in which, though vision is perfect while the sun is above the horizon, the patient is incapable of seeing by the aid of artificial light. The eye presents no external appearance of mal-organization, and the rationale of this peculiarity has never been explained.

Hemicrania.—Pain confined to one half of the head. It is always intermittent; sometimes continuing only while the sun is above the horizon, and is then called *Sun-pain*. It is symptomatic of that condition of diseased liver which accompanies intermittent fever, and is to be cured by restoring the function of that viscus.

Hemiopia.—Depraved vision in which the person sees only one half of an object.

Hemiphonia.—Great weakness of voice. It may result from malconformation of the respiratory apparatus, debility of the respiratory laryngeal muscles, or obstruction in the brain, lungs, or liver.

Hemiplegia.—Palsy of one side of the body. See Paralysis.

Hemorrhage—Bleeding. See Hæmorrhagia.

Hemorrhoids.—See Hæmorrhois.

Hepatalgia.—Pain in the Liver.

Hepathæmorrhagia.—Hemorrhage of the Liver. It sometimes occurs in putrid fevers.

HEPATITIS.—Inflammation of the Liver. *Acute* inflammation of the liver is a rare affection in this latitude, though common in tropical climates. It is known by acute and constant pain in the right side, shooting to the back and shoulders, increased on pressure; difficulty of lying on the right side, short breath, cough, jaundice, and general fever. Tepid enemas to free the bowels, the wet-girdle constantly, with tepid ablutions to the whole surface, or the wet-sheet pack, as the degree of the external heat may demand, constitute the plan of treatment. *Chronic Hepatitis*, which is one of the forms of "liver complaint" so prevalent in this country, is known by a less degree of the above local symptoms, and the absence of fever. The proper medicinal appliances are the wet-girdle a part of each day, or, in cold weather, during the night, hip-baths—75° to 85°—once or twice a day, the wet-sheet pack once or twice a week, the dripping-sheet or sponge-bath each morning on rising, providing the external temperature is sufficient; otherwise, the dry-rubbing sheet a part of the time instead of the wet; abdominal manipulations, or "Swedish Movements," and a very plain vegetarian, and rather abstemious dietary. Milk, grease, and hard water are specially objectionable in this disease.

HEPATIZATION.—A state of the lungs in which they are engorged with effused matter, so that they become impervious to air.

HEPATOCELE.—Hernia of the Liver. Protrusions of the liver from enlargement of the organ, or poison, or injuries to the walls of the abdomen, have been so termed.

HEPATOGASTROCHOLOSIS.—A formidable technicality which has been applied to "bilious" and "gastric" fevers.

HEPATOPATHIA.—Disease of the Liver.

HEPATOSCIRRHUS.—Scirrhus or Cancer of the Liver.

HERNIA.—Any tumor formed by the displacement of a viscus, or of some portion of a viscus, which has escaped from its natural cavity by some aperture. Herniæ are divided into *encephalic, thoracic,* and *abdominal.*

The medication is mainly surgical ; and for the various forms and manner of treatment, we must refer to the standard works on surgery. What is called the *radical cure* of hernia, consists in maintaining for several weeks that degree of pressure which will excite adhesive inflammation. In some cases several months are required to effect a cure.

HERNIA, HUMORALIS.—This term has been applied to inflammation of the testicle.

HERPES.—Tetters, Fret. A vesicular eruption. The vesicles appear in distinct but irregular clusters on an inflamed base, and pass through a regular course of increase, maturation, and decline, in ten days to two weeks. The affection is attended with heat, pain, and considerable constitutional feverishness. Some authors have three varieties, the *Miliary*, *Vesicular*, and *Eroding*. The cause is acrid bile or retained effete matters, and the process of cure is simply one of purification. A daily wet-sheet pack or tepid ablution, two or three times a day, are all the bathing processes required.

HICCOUGH, HICCUP.—Singultus. A clonic spasm of the respiratory muscles, which arrests the air in the windpipe, while the diaphragm contracts, occasioning a peculiar sound. It is symptomatic of fatigue, debility, or obstruction, and in low fevers is indicative of danger. It can generally be arrested by bits of ice, fomentations to the abdomen, and in many cases by fixing the mind intently on any subject or object.

HIDDEN SEIZURES.—An awkward term employed by MARSHALL HALL to designate obscure forms of epileptic spasms.

HILON.—Hilum, Hilus. Terms applied to a small blackish tumor, formed by the protrusion of the iris through an opening in the transparent cornea.

HIP-DISEASE.—See Coxarum Morbus.

HIPPANTHROPIA.—A variety of melancholy, in which the patient believes himself changed to a horse.

HIPPURIA.—Excess of hippuric acid in the urine.

HIPPUS.—Morbid twinkling of the eyes.

HIRSUTIES.—Trichosis, Hairiness. Growth of hairs on parts normally destitute, as in bearded women. Various caustics— "depilatories"—of which preparations of iron, arsenic, quick-silver, potash, etc., are the chief ingredients, have been employed to remove them.

HIRUDOLISMUS.—Hirudo, the Leech. We coin this technicality to express the process of abstracting the life-blood by means of leeches. When the Hygienic method of purifying the blood is fully recognized by physicians, they will see a better use for blood than feeding it to leeches.

HIVES.—Hyves. This term has been variously applied to *Croup, Urticaria,* and *Varicella.* In Scotland it means any eruption of the skin arising from an internal cause.

HOARSENESS.—This results from congestion, thickening, or ulceration of the mucous membrane of the trachea, larynx, throat or nose, or from obstruction of the lungs, enlargement of the liver, weakness of the abdominal muscles, and various other causes.

HOB-NAIL LIVER.—Cirrhosis of the Liver.

HOMESICKNESS.—See Nostalgia.

HORDEOLUM.—Stye. A small inflammatory tumor, of the nature of a boil, on the free edge of the eyelids. The skillful application of a frigorific in the incipient stage, will arrest it at once; otherwise the part may be frequently bathed with water of the temperature that is most agreeable.

HORNY EXCRESCENCES.—Cornua, Horns. Excrescences in shape resembling the horns of animals, which occasionally form on some part of the skin. They sometimes grow to several inches in length. They should be removed by excision or ligature, and the part from which they spring deeply cauterized with nitric acid or sulphate of zinc.

HORRIPILATION.—Horror. The general chilliness which precedes violent fevers, and accompanied with bristling of hairs of the body.

HORSE CRUST.—*Crusta genu equinæ.*

HOSPITAL GANGRENE.—Putrid or Malignant Ulcer. Gangrene occurring in ulcers or wounds in hospitals. It is caused mainly by vitiated air.

HUMOR.—Every fluid of an organized body is called a *humor*, as blood, chyle, lymph, etc. *Morbid humor* means any depraved fluid or secretion. The *Humoral Pathology*—Humorism—is the doctrine that the fluids are the primary seat of disease, or primarily affected in disease, the affection or disease of the solids being secondary and consequential. The *Nervous Pathology* is the reverse of this.

HUMP.—Hunch, Gibber, Tuber. A prominence formed by a deviation of the bones of the trunk from the normal position. The spine may be curved backwards, forwards, or laterally. Curvatures are the result of injuries, relaxation of the abdominal and dorsal muscles, or of the scrofulous diathesis.

HYDARTHRUS.—See Hydrarthrus.

HYDATID.—Hydrocystis, Encysted tumors containing an aqueous fluid, or vesicles developed with organs, but without adhering to their tissue. They have been found in the uterus, ovaries, liver, and various other parts of the body.

HYDATOCELE.—See Hydrocele.

HYDEROS.—Hydrops. See Anasarca.

HYDRADENITIS.—Inflammation of a lymphatic gland.

HYDRÆMIA.—See Hydrœmia.

HYDRARGYRIA.—Mercurial Eczema; Mercurial Leprosy. Eczema induced by mercurial poison. For the treatment, see Eczema, Mercuriale.

HYDRARGYRIASIS. — Mercurialismus ; Poisoning by mercury; Mercurial Fever. Authors have noted no less than *fifty-one* distinct diseases which are occasioned by mercurial medicines. The time cannot be far distant when physicians and people will look back with horror on this most absurd and outrageously abominable practice.

HYDRARGYROSIS.—Eczema Mercuriale.

HYDRARGYRO-STOMATITIS.—Salivation, which see.

HYDRARTHRUS.—Hydrarthrosis, Articular Dropsy, White Swelling. It may affect any one of the joints, but most commonly affects that of the knee. Scrofulous children are almost always the subjects of it. It may consist in swelling and softening of the soft parts and ligaments, or in ulceration of the articular extremities of the bones.

In the treatment, the part should be constantly enveloped with cold wet cloths, covered with dry, and frequently renewed. This practice should be continued so long as there is preternatural heat in the part, after which gentle showering or douching, followed by gentle friction, should be persevered in until the restoration is complete. The general system must be treated according to its condition—all the processes of purification and invigoration practicable being resorted to. The diet should be strictly vegetarian, largely frugivorous, and milk, butter and cheese rigidly prohibited. A daily tepid ablution, with the wet-sheet pack once a week, will usually be all that is required in the way of general bathing.

HYDROCEPHALUS.—See Hydrocephalus Internus.

HYDROÆMIA.—Anæmia, which see.

HYDROCELE.—Dropsy of the Scrotum. A collection of serous fluid in the areolar texture of the scrotum, or in some of the coverings of the testicle or spermatic chord. The collection most frequently occurs in the envelope of the testicle, the *tunica vaginalis testis.* It may be distinguished from sarcoma or other tumors by its semi-transparency, and by the oblong shape of the tumor; also by its being greater below than above. In the incipient or early stage it can often be removed by means of persevering friction and the fountain or spray bath, and one or two sitz-baths—70° to 80°—daily, in connection with an abstemious dietary, and such general bathing as the general health requires. But if these measures fail, the radical cure consists in puncturing the tumor with a trocar, evacuating the water, and injecting through the camula of the trocar, some irritating substance to excite adhesive inflammation. Wine, diluted alcohol, solution of sulphate of zinc, and the tincture of iodine have been employed successfully. The latter is perhaps the most convenient and efficacious.

HYDROCEPHALUS.—Water in the Head; Dropsy of the Brain. Medical authors distinguish it into *Chronic*, *External*, and *Internal*, or *Acute*. *Chronic Hydrocephalus* is often congenital, and generally fatal. The fluid gradually accumulates in the cavities of the brain, distending the organ and separating the sutures. It is one of the numerous manifestations of scrofula, and little can be done in the way of medication, except keeping the head cool, the feet warm, the bowels free, the skin open by means of tepid ablutions and gentle friction. *External Hydrocephalus* is a mere infiltration into the subcutaneous cellular tissue of the cranium, and may easily be removed by cold applications. *Internal Hydrocephalus* is a misnomer. The disease so called consists in scrofulous inflammation of the membranes of the brain, and has been called *Tubercular Meningitis*. The first symptoms are, feverishness with headache, intolerance of light and sound, and delirium; these are succeeded, in the second stage, by moaning, dilated pupil, squinting, starting, and crying out as if in distress; in the third or last stage the child is comatose or stupid, and affected more or less with paralysis and convulsions. The progress of the disease is rapid, and usually terminates in death in from three days to three weeks.

Treatment can seldom avail, except when commenced within the first stage. The whole surface should be frequently sponged with tepid water, so as to keep the heat down to the normal standard; a cold wet cloth must be kept on the head, and very frequently changed, so long as the local heat is preternatural; the temperature of the room must be kept at all times mild and uniform, and ventilation carefully attended to.

HYDRODERMA.—Anasarca.

HYDROMANIA.—A term applied to *Pellagra*, in which the patient feels a strong propensity to drown himself.

HYDROMETRA.—Hydrops Uteri, Dropsy of the Womb. A

rare disease, and doubted altogether by some authors. The symptoms are said to be, a circumscribed protuberance of the hypogastrium, with obscure fluctuation, progressively enlarging, without ischury or pregnancy.

HYDROPHOBIA.—Rabies; Canine Madness. This disease may be developed in animals by whatever overheats and inflames the blood, and befouls the secretions and excretions; after which it may be communicated to other animals or persons through the media of the saliva and bronchial mucus. The chief symptoms are, sense of dryness and constriction in the throat; excessive thirst; difficult deglutition; aversion for and horror at the sight of brilliant objects, and of liquids; flushed face; great irritability; frothy saliva; grinding of the teeth, etc. Though the virus may remain for months in the system before the disease is manifest, the patient seldom lives more than four or five days after its commencement. So far as we can learn from the testimony of medical books and journals, the malady has been uniformly fatal under drug treatment. Cases of recovery, however, are given in which patients have recovered when no drugs of any kind were administered.

The direct indication is to favor the elimination of the poison in all possible ways, and soothe the nervous irritation as much as possible. The warm-bath followed by the tepid ablution, the prolonged tepid half-bath, or the wet-sheet pack, when the patient can be controlled, are the best of the bathing processes. Pieces of ice can often be taken with comfort and benefit, when water cannot be swallowed without exciting distressing spasms.

Preventive measures should always be resorted to, when practicable. The bitten part should be excised or cauterized. Any drug capable of immediately disorganizing the injured part, so as to prevent the absorption of the virus, will be efficient; but the more potent the application the better. Nitric acid, caustic potash, quick lime, ammonia, etc., have been employed successfully.

HYDROPTHALMIA.—Dropsy of the Eye. An affection caused by an abnormal quantity of the aqueous or vitreous humor, or of both. Children are most subject to it. It is usually connected with a scrofulous diathesis, and almost invariably preceded by constipated bowels. The most important part of the remedial plan is a correct dietary..

HYDROPS.—Dropsy. An abnormal collection of a serous fluid, in the areolar tissue, or in any cavity of the body. When the areolar tissue of the whole body is more or less filled with fluid, the affection is termed *Anasarca*, or *Leucophlegmatia;* and when this variety is local or partial it is called *Œdema*. When the fluid is enclosed in a sac or cyst, the disease is termed *Encysted Dropsy*. As the action of the skin and kidneys is defective in all forms of dropsical affections, the direct indication in all cases is to restore the functions of those organs. The treatment applicable to the various forms of dropsy is mentioned under their respective heads.

HYDRORACHIS.—Dropsy of the spine; Spina Bifida. An effusion of serum, forming a soft, frequently transparent tumor, constituted of the membranes of the spinal marrow. When the affection is congenital, the posterior walls of the vertebral canal are wanting to a certain extent, from which point the tumor projects backwards. It is seldom or never curable.

HYDROTHORAX.—Dropsy of the Chest. Idiopathic hydrothorax is extremely rare.. When symptomatic, it indicates extreme obstruction or exhaustion, and is, hence, in a great majority of cases, incurable., We have, however, cured a few cases in their early stages. Short breath, frequent small pulse, sense of weight or oppression in the chest, and swelling of the lower extremities, are the principal symptoms. Tepid ablutions with gentle but thorough and persevering friction to the whole surface, and a spare, plain dietary, are the essentials of the treatment. Milk and sugar must be abstained from, and every article of food should be solid, dry, and well masticated.

HYDRURESIS.—See Diabetes.

HYPERACUSIS.—Morbid sensibility of the organ of hearing. It exists in many forms of fever.

HYPERÆMIA.—Local Congestion.   Preternatural determination of blood to a part.

HYPERAPHIA.—Excessive Acuteness of Touch.

HYPERAPHRODISIA.—Inordinate Venereal Passion.

HYPERCARDIA.—Hypertrophy of the Heart.

HYPERCATHARSIS.—Excessive Purgation.

HYPEREMESIS.—Excessive Vomiting after an Emetic.

HYPERSARCOMA.—Fungosity on Ulcerated Parts.

HYPERSTEMIA.—The Entonic Diathesis, Inflammatory Fever.

HYPERTONIA.—This is defined in the medical dictionaries to be, "excessive tone in parts;" but such a condition cannot exist. We might as well talk of *excessive health*. It means *active* inflammation, or a vigorous determination of blood to the part—the opposite of *passive* inflammation, or atony.

HYPERTROPHY.—Abdominal Increase of Bulk.

HYPNOTISM.—Somnambulism, Animal Magnetism.

HYPOCHONDRIASIS.—Hypo, Spleen, Vapors, Low Spirits. A condition of dysyepsia or liver complaint, in which the patient is constantly troubled on the subject of his health, with a continual succession of uneasy feelings and mental illusions. Some authors locate the seat of this malady in the brain, but I think it will always be found in the digestive apparatus. In managing this class of invalids occupation is of much importance.

HYPONOMAS.—A deep fistula or ulcer.

HYPONYCHON.—Effusion of blood under a nail.

HYPOPYON.—Pyosis; Abscesses of the Eye. Small abscesses between the layers of the cornea ; also collections of purulent matter in the chambers of the eye. Subdue the pain and morbid heat with cold applications, and then, if necessary, puncture the cornea and evacuate the pus.

HYPERSARCOSIS.—A Wart.

HYSTERALGIA.—Irritable Uterus; Pain in the Uterus, Uterine Neuralgia. It is a frequent accompaniment of dysmenorrhœa and chronic inflammation.

Hysteria.—It occurs in paroxysms of alternate fits of laughing and crying, with a sensation (Globus Hystericus) as if a ball ascended to the neck, producing a feeling of strangulation. It is not confined to the female, for irritable, nervous men are occasionally the subjects of it. It is often connected with menstrual disorder. The paroxysm may be relieved by cold applications to the head and face, warm applications to the feet, and abdominal fomentations. To prevent a recurrence of the fits, it is necessary to restore the general health. The remedial plan should embrace the utmost tranquillity of mind and body, and, if practicable, agreeable occupation or amusements.

Hysterocele.—Hernia of the Womb. A rare disease; but the uterus may protrude through the lower part of the linea alba, or through the inguinal or the crural canal.

Hysteromania.—See Nymphomania.

Hystriciasis.—A morbid condition, in which the hairs stand erect, like the quills of the porcupine.

Ichor.—Sanies, Foul Pus, Virus, Sordes. A thin, acrid, watery discharge from foul ulcers.

Ichthyosis.—Fish-skin, Porcupine Disease. A dry, scaly, and, in some cases, almost horny texture of the skin. Obstruction of the cutaneous pores, and foulness of blood, are the causes, and bathing, friction, and a pure dietary, are the remedies.

Icthyosis Pellagra.—See Pellagra.

Icthyosis Sebacea.—An incrustation of a concrete substance upon the surface of the epidermis.

Icteric Fever.—See Fever, Icteric.

Icterus.—Bilious Dyscrasy, Yellows, Jaundice. This affection is characterized by yellowness of the skin and eyes, light-colored feces, and high-colored urine. Its immediate cause is torpidity of the liver. A tepid ablution daily, the wet-sheet pack weekly, the wet-girdle a part of each day, when the external temperature is sufficient, and one or two hip-baths daily, are the proper bathing appliances. Abdominal manipulations are often indispensable; the dietary can scarcely be too plain. Hydro-Electrical baths are adapted to low states of the circulation. Milk, grease, and fine flour should be abstained from, and the patient should carefully avoid drinking hard water.

ICTERUS ALBUS.—Chlorosis.

ICTERUS INFANTUM.—Yellow Gum, Jaundice of Infants.

ICTERUS MELAS.—Melœna, Black Jaundice.

ICTERUS SATURNINUS.—Jaundice occasioned by lead poisoning.

ICTUS.—A Stroke or Blow. See *Coup de Soleil*.

IDIOPATHIA.—A Primary Disease.

IDIOSYNCRASY.—A peculiarity of constitution, in which one person is affected very differently from the majority by certain agents and influences. Thus, some persons faint at the sight of blood; others cannot bear milk, butter, or cheese, shell-fish, etc., without disgust, distress, or sickness.

IDIOTISM.—Fatuity. It is often congenital, but may supervene on mania, melancholy, and other maladies. Many children are born hopelessly demented or imbecile, because one or both parents were in a debauched, drunken, morbid, exhausted, feverish, or inflammatory condition at the time of conception. Excessive bleeding has occasionally reduced adults to perpetual idiotism.

IGNIS.—Fire.

IGNIS CALIDUS.—Acute *Passive* Inflammation about to degenerate into gangrene.

IGNIS FRIGIDUS.—A Cold Fire. See Sphacelus.

IGNIS PERSICUS.—Erysipelas.

IGNIS SACER.—Herpes, Erysipelas.

IGNIS SYLVATICUS.—Crusta Lactea of Infants.

ILEITIS.—Inflammation of the Ileum. See Enteritis.

ILEO-CHOLOSIS.—Bilious Diarrhœa.

ILEO-COLITIS.—See Enteritis.

ILEUS.—Iliac Passion; Spasmodic Colic. See Colic, Convulsive.

ILLEGITIMATE, OR BASTARD.—This term is applied to fevers and inflammations whose paroxysms are extraordinary or anomalous.

ILLOSIS.—Strabismus.

ILLUSION.—Hallucination.

IMPERFORATION.—Absence of a natural aperture, as of the mouth, anus, vulva, nostrils, etc.

IMPETIGO.—Running Scall or Tetter. This term is applied to a variety of cutaneous diseases, and to some forms of cachexia. See Psoriasis.

IMPOSTHUME.—Abscess.

IMPOTENCE.—Impuissance. Loss of power over one or more members; usually applied to the sexual organs. When the constitutional vigor is exhausted there is, of course, no remedy. In other cases all that is required, and all that can be done, is to restore the general health. The stimulants and excitants advertised by the quacks, as Essences of Life, Rejuvenators, Invigorators, etc., etc., are only intended to rob the unfortunate and despairing. They injure all and cure none.

IMPOVERISHED.—Poor Blood. The idea that preparations of iron, arsenic, cod-liver oil, blood-gravy, alcoholic liquors, etc., can enrich poor, or rectify impure blood, is one of the most preposterously absurd fantasies that ever possessed the minds of intelligent beings. Good food, fresh air, pure water, and proper exercise are the only "blood-foods" that nature owns or blesses.

IMPUISSANCE.—See Impotence.

INANITION.—Exhaustion for want of nourishment. The feverishness which attends starvation or innutrition has been called the "Hectic of inanition."

INCARCERATION.—A condition in hernia in which the sac is constricted about its neck, so that it cannot be returned to its

8*

place without difficulty. The term is sometimes used in the sense of *strangulation*.

INCARNATION.—Growth of flesh, or granulations.

INCUBATION.—In pathology, this term is applied to the period which elapses between the introduction of a morbific agent and the manifestation of the consequent disease, as in small-pox, measles, rabies, etc.

INCUBUS.—Nightmare. This affection is almost always caused by indigestion, or an overloaded stomach. It consists in a sensation of distressing weight at the epigastrium during sleep, without the power to move, speak or breathe—the patient at length awakening in terror. Avoid the causes.

INCUBUS VIGILANTIUM.—Daymare. A sense of pressure over the abdomen, with frequent and laborious respiration, occurring during wakefulness..

INDICATION.—In nosology, a symptom; in pathology, the direct object to be accomplished by remedial measures: Thus, in apoplexy the indication is, to determine the blood *from* the brain; in cholera, to determine circulation *to* the skin.

INDIGESTION.—See Dyspepsia.

INDISPOSITION.—Any slight sickness.

INDOLENT.—An epithet applied to painless and inactive tumors and ulcers.

INDURATION.—Hardness of tissue, the result of inflammation.

INEBRIATION.—Intoxication, Temulentia. There are all degrees of this affection, from a slight *fuddlement*—exhilaration—to the apoplectic stupor or dead-drunkenness. The treatment is the same as for apoplexy. The remedy is "*teetotalism.*"

INESIS, INETHMOS.—Cenosis.

INFANTILE FEVER.—See Fever, Infantile Remittent.

INFECTIOUS DISEASES.—Diseases which are caused by the application or ingeneration of some animal venom or virus, as syphilis, hydrophobia, etc. The term infection is often employed synonymously with contagion, but this strictly applies to formites, malaria, and other "morbid poisons" which are communicated through the medium of the atmosphere.

INFILTRATION.—Effusion. Accumulation of any fluid in the areolar tissue.

INFIRMITY.—Any morbid condition ; in contradistinction to morbid *action*, which constitutes the essence of disease.

INFLAMMATION.—The diagnostic symptoms of inflammation are, heat, pain, redness, and swelling ; add to these *fever* and we have *Visceral Inflammation*, as cephalitis, pneumonitis, gastritis, etc. The fever accompanying visceral inflammations may be entonic or atonic, inflammatory or typhoid, as in simple fevers. The fever, it should be understood, is a part of the disease, and not symptomatic, as the books have it. Endless confusion in pathology and therapeutics, and not a little of the fatal practice extant are the results of this error. For example, in typhoid pneumonia, medical authors cannot agree whether the fever, (which is of the typhus or typhoid form) or whether the inflammation of the lungs, is the primary disease. Neither is true. Both the local and the constitutional affection are parts of one and the same disease. When the constitutional affection is *atonic fever* the local affection will be *erysipelatous, erythematic, asthenic, adynamic, passive*, etc., *inflammation ;* and when the constitutional affection is *entonic fever*, the local affection will be *phlegmonous* or *adhesive inflammation*, and *vice versa*. A world of confusion would be prevented, and an awful extent of malpractice would be obviated, if this distinction would be recognized by the profession. As it is, those physicians who regard the inflammation as primary and the fever as secondary, direct the strength of their treatment to the reduction of the inflammation, by bleeding, leeching, blistering, narcotics, and antiphlogistics, though these measures confessedly increase the constitutional debility, and aggravate the typhoid state. And on the other hand, those who regard the fever as primary and the inflammation as secondary, pursue the opposite practice—opium, alcohol, spirits nitre, turpentine, etc.—though injurious to the state of the lungs. Both prac-

tices are wrong, as both theories are erroneous. For several
centuries the medical profession has been debating the question, whether inflammation is an *increased* or a *decreased* action
of the parts ; and they are no nearer a solution of the problem
now than when the discussion was commenced. It is neither.
It is simply *irregular, abnormal* action. It is *morbid* action as is a
fever, or any other disease, properly so called. It is inflammation when there is disproportionate accumulation of blood
(congestion) in some part, attended with heat, redness, pain,
and swelling. When the morbid action (remedial effort) disturbs the whole organism, without the existence of the above
local condition, the disease is *fever*. In some visceral inflammations the fever may be entonic or atonic, as pneumonitis,
gastritis, enteritis, etc., and in others it is always atonic, as
diptheria, croup, influenza, dysentery, etc. The *type* of the
fever of visceral inflammation is always *continued*. *Chronic
inflammation* is always characterized by the absence of fever at
the outset, as in consumption, hip-disease, dyspepsia, etc., and
when fever supervenes in the course of the disease, it is of the
remittent type, and is termed *hectic*. The notion that the type
and diathesis of the inflammation depend on the particular
tissue which is the seat of it, is among the numerous and unfortunate errors of the medical profession ; and not only unfortunate but disastrous, for it has been the death of millions of
the human race. They depend solely on the condition of the
patient, whether gross, feeble, or vigorous, as I have explained
under the head of fever.

INFLAMMATION, BOWELS, OF THE.—See Enteritis.

INFLAMMATION, BRAIN, OF THE.—See Cephalitis.

INFLAMMATION, EAR, OF THE.—See Otitis.

INFLAMMATION, EYE, OF THE.—Se Opthalmitis.

INFLAMMATION, HEART, OF THE.—See Carditis.

INFLAMMATION, KIDNEYS, OF THE.—See Nephritis.

IMFLAMMATION, LARYNX, OF THE.—See Laryngitis.

INFLAMMATION, LIVER, OF THE.—See Hepatitis.

INFLAMMATION, LUNGS, OF THE.—See Pneumonitis.

INFLAMMATION, PERITONEUM, OF THE.—See Peritonitis.

INFLAMMATION, PLEURA, OF THE.—See Pleuritis.

INFLAMMATION, SPLEEN, OF THE.—See Spenitis.

INFLAMMATION, STOMACH, OF THE.—See Gastritis.

INFLAMMATION, TESTES, OF THE.—See Orchitis.

INFLAMMATION, THROAT, OF THE.—See Stomatitis.

INFLAMMATION, TONSILS, OF THE.—See Tonsillitis.

INFLAMMATION, VAGINA, OF THE.—See Vaginitis.

INFLAMMATION, UTERUS, OF THE.—See Metritis.

INFLUENZA.—Epidemic Catarrh. An inflammatory affection involving the mucous membrane of the nose and windpipe and its bronchial ramifications. It usually occurs epidemically, and often extends over a large area of territory. The fever is of the low or typhoid character, attended with sweating, sometimes profuse, and the chief local symptoms are cough, thirst, watery eyes, and great sense of oppression in the chest. The debility is often extreme, though the disease, aside from bad medication, is one of little or no danger.

INSANITY.—Unsound Mind, Deranged Intellect, Delirium, Mania. The term is generic and includes all varieties of mental alienation.

INSENSIBILITY.—Anæsthesia. Loss or absence of Feeling.

INSOMNIA.—Morbid Vigilance, Sleeplessness. It indicates determination to the brain, or some disturbing influence within or without. It is a frequent symptom in fevers, and is often one of the most troublesome complications of dyspeptics.

INTEMPERANCE.—Usually applied to the immoderate and habitual use of intoxicating drinks, but equally applicable to excessive alimentation. Gluttony is, throughout the civilized world, as great an evil as intemperance; indeed, improper dietetic habits are the chief causes of that morbid appetite which leads to the use of alcoholic beverages.

INTERMISSION.—The interval between two paroxysms of in termittent fever. The pulse is said to *intermit* when one or more beats is wanting in a given number—a state of pulse very common with dyspeptics.

INTERMITTENT FEVER.—See Fever, Intermittent.

INTERTRIGO.—Chafing, Fret, Erosions of the Skin. Red excoriations which occur in consequence of the friction of parts. Washing the part frequently with cold water and dusting it with flour or hair-powder will readily cure them, if the general health is duly attended to.

INTOXICATION.—The disturbance of the bodily and mental functions occasioned by the use of alcoholic liquors. Opium, tobacco, tea, coffee, and many other articles induce various forms and degrees of intoxication.

INTUMESCENCE.—Swelling, Tumefaction ; Augmentation of size in a part.

INTUSSUSCEPTION.—The introduction of one part of the intestinal tube into another. In most cases it is the upper portion of the small intestine which is intussuscepted. See Colic, Convulsive.

IODINISM.—When Iodine has been given in large doses, or long continued, it often occasions an exhausting colliquative diarrhœa, with rapid emaciation and death. In many cases the male testes, and in others the female breasts, are almost entirely absorbed.

IONTHUS.—Violent eruption, Varus. A tubercular tumor of the face.

IRITIS.—Inflammation of the Iris. With the usual symptoms of inflammation there are tooth-like processes projecting into the pupil, while this is irregularly contracted. For treatment, see Opthalmitis.

IRRITATION.—Erythisnus. Morbid circulation and sensibility, without the diagnostic symptoms of inflammation.

IRRITATIVE FEVER.—General Irritation.

ISCHIOCELE.—Ischiatic Hernia.

ISCHURIA.—Stoppage of Urine. Inability to discharge the urine. It is applied both to the suppression of the excretion and to its accumulation in the bladder. When the urine is retained, if alternate hot and cold applications do not succeed in exciting the expulsive action of the bladder, the catheter must be employed. The necessity for this process may be known by the hard, painful, and increasing tumefaction at the lower part of the abdomen. When the excretion does not take place, the remedy consists in restoring the action of the kidneys.

ISTHMITIS.—Inflammation of the Fauces. Gurgling with cold water, holding ice in the mouth, and the application of a cold wet cloth around the throat, are the local appliances.

ITCH.—Psora, Scabies, Scratch. A variety of cutaneous eruptions are called itch, as Cow-pox, Psoriasis, Bakers' Itch, Sycosis, Barbers' Itch, etc. But the *real* itch is produced by an insect of the genus acarus, which burrows under the skin, exciting inflammation with intolerable itching. Various poisons, as mercurial preparations, sulphur, iodine, turpentine, hellebore, and tobacco, will destroy it; but we have never yet failed with thorough ablution and persevering friction. See Psoria.

ITIS.—A suffix denoting inflammation.

JACTATION.—Extreme Anxiety, or Excessive Restlessness. A symptom of many serious diseases.

JAUNDICE.—Icterus, which see.

JAW DISEASE.—Ulceration of the Lower-Jaw, by Phosphorus. Those who are exposed to its fumes in the manufacture of lucifer and congreve matches are subject to it.

JECORIS VOMICA.—See Hepatitis.

JEJUNITIS.—Inflammation of the Jejunum. See Enteritis.

JERKS.—See Mania, Dancing.

JIGGER.—See Chique.

JUNGLE FEVER.—A Remittent of India.

KINCOUGH, KINDCOUGH.—See Pertussis.

KING'S EVIL.—Scrofula.

KINK IN THE HEAD.—Insanity.

KIRRHONOSIS, KIRRHOSIS.—Cirrhosis.

KLEPTOMANIA, KLOPEMANIA.—Insanity with a propensity to steal.

KNEE SCAB.—Crusta genu equinæ.

KYANOSIS.—Cyanopathy.

KYLLOSIS.—Congenital Distortion of the Foot. Talipes, Clubfoot.

KYSTHITIS.—See Vaginitis.

LABORIOUS.—Parturition and Respiration are said to be *laborious* when performed with great difficulty.

LACERATION.—Rupture, Dilaceration. Breach made by tearing and rending.

LAGOPHTHALMIA.—Hare's Eye: A retraction of the upper eyelid so that it does not cover the globe of the eye during sleep.

LANCINATING.—Shooting or darting pains, as in cancers, are so termed.

LANGOR.—Sense of Weariness.

LARDACEOUS.—Alterations of the textures so that they resemble lard in aspect and consistency.

LARYNGISMUS STRIDULUS.—Asthma Thymicum, Spasmodic Quinsy, Spasm of the Glottis, Child-Crowing, Spasmodic Croup, Spurious Croup. A disease, mostly of infants, characterized by intervals of suspended respiration, great difficulty of breathing, especially on swallowing or crying, and frequently ending in a fit of suffocation with convulsions. It is a spasmodic affection of the respiratory and articulating muscles, induced by some irritating agent, or by obstruction in the alimentary canal. Fomentations to the abdomen, warm foot-baths, and cold applications to the head and neck, are the remedies.

LARYNGITIS.—Inflammation of the Larynx. The symptoms resemble those of croup, but may be distinguished by the absence of the sonorous inspiration, and by pain upon pressing the larynx. Cold and wet cloths around the throat, bits of ice held in the mouth, or frequent sips of iced-water, with such attention to general bathing as the febrile symptoms demand, will speedily reduce it.

Chronic Laryngitis is a form of consumption, which see.

Lax.—Diarrhœa.

Lead Poisoning.—Molybdosis, Morbus Plumbeus. See Colic, Metallic.

Leaping Ague.—See Mania, Dancing.

Lepidosarcoma.—A fleshy tumor covered with scales.

Lepidosis.—Scaly diseases.

Lepidosis Ichthyiasis.—Horny Excrescences.

Lepra.—Leprosy. The varieties of this disease are very numerous, as *White, Black, Common*, etc., each comprehending several sub-varieties. The leprosy of the Jews consisted of shining patches, on which the hair turned white and silky, the skin losing its sensibility. It was incurable. The leprosy of the Arabs was a form of Elephantiasis. That of the Greeks is characterized by scaly patches of different sizes and of a circular form. Lepra is endemic in Egypt, in Java, and in certain parts of Norway and Sweden. All varieties of this disease are but the outside manifestations of foul blood and exhausted nerves, and tell the story of gross diet, inattention to personal cleanliness, or dissipation in some of its multitudinous forms. I have seen several marked cases of leprosy in this city, and at "Hygeian Home," the result of accumulated acrid and putrescent bilious matter in the system.

Tepid ablutions, with as much exercise in the open air as the patient can take short of great fatigue, and a simple, abstemious, vegetarian dietary, constitute the remedial plan.

Lesion.—Disorder, Derangement. Any morbid structural or functional change.

Lethargy.—A state of stupor from which it is impossible to arouse the patient, except momentarily. It is always a symptomatic affection.

Leucæmia.—Deficiency of coloring matter of the blood.

LEUCOCYTHÆMIA.—Superabundance of white corpuscles in the blood; a condition said to be accompanied with enlargement of the spleen, liver, and lymphatic glands,

LEUCOMA.—Leucosis, Albugo, Ephelotes. Opacity of the cornea.

LEUCONECROSIS.—A form of dry Gangrene.

LEUCOPHLEGMASIA.—A dropsical habit. General Dropsy.

LEUCORRHŒA.—Fluor Albus, Whites, Uterine Catarrh, Vaginitis. An excretion of white, yellowish, or greenish mucus from the lining membrane of the female genital organs. It is a result of inflammation. It is attended with pain, heat, a sense of weight or heaviness in the loins, and when severe, with a sense of burning or scalding in urinating. It may be important in some cases to know that the female who has leucorrhœa with a very acrid discharge, may communicate to the male, in the act of copulation, a similar morbid condition. This has been sometimes mistaken for that form of venereal disease called gonorrhœa. Of the many causes of this very common malady, none is so general and so efficient as constipation of the bowels; and hence nothing in the plan of medication can be more indispensable than a strict dietary. Milk, grease, and condiments of all kinds should be rigidly abstained from, and fine flour, starchy preparations, puddings, etc., should be avoided. Tepid hip-baths, the wet-girdle, and vaginal injections, the temperature and frequency being determined more or less by the temperature and debility of the patient, are the special "hydropathic" appliances. Fresh air and moderate exercise are not to be overlooked; and when constipation is very considerable, or the abdominal muscles greatly relaxed, manipulations, or the Swedish Movements, are excellent auxilliaries.

Leucorrhœa is often connected with prolapsus, or other displacements of the uterus, and this condition must be duly regarded in directing the exercises and manipulations.

LICHEN.—Scabies Sicca, Exormia. A general term including several species of cutaneous affections, among which are

Prickly Heat, Summer Rash, Nettle Rash, etc. Tepid ablutions, and a spare, simple dietary, are all the treatment they require.

LIENTERY.—Laxness of the Bowels, Dyspeptic Diarrhœa. Frequent liquid evacuations, the food only partially digested. Treat the dyspeptic condition.

LIMOCTONIA.—Starvation ; Suicide by Hunger.

LIMOSIS.—Stomach Disease ; Indigestion.

LIPAROCELE.—Fatty Tumor of the Scrotum.

LIPOMA.—A Fatty Tumor.

LIPOSIS.—See Polysarcia.

LIPPITUDO.—Blear-Eye, Gleme, Lema, Gramia. A gummy state of the eyelids from a copious excretion of the sebaceous follicles, the result of chronic inflammation.

LITHIA, LITHIASIS.—Calculous cachexia. The formation of calculous concretions; gravel, or stone in the human body. The term is also applied to an affection of the eyelids in which small, hard, stone-like concretions form on their edges.

LIVER DISEASE.—See Jaundice, Hepatitis, and Cirrhosis.

LIVER-GROWN.—Chronic enlargement of the organ.

LIVER, HOB-NAIL.—Cirrhosis of the organ.

LIVER, NUTMEG.—Tuberculation of the liver ; the effect of intemperance. The terms, *gin-liver, gin-drinkers' liver,* and *whisky-liver,* are also applied to this condition.

LIVER SPOT.—Chloasma, Cirrhosis.

LOCHIA.—The Cleanings. The serous and sanguineous discharge which follows delivery. When this discharge is suddenly suppressed by cold or other causes, there is difficult breathing, headache, or "rush of blood" to the head, and often delirium. It should be promptly restored by means of warm hip-baths, fomentations to the abdomen, hot foot-baths, etc.

LOCHIORRHAGIA.—Excessive Lochial Discharge. Cold applications to the abdomen, cool vaginal injections, and enemas of cold water will check it.

LOCKED-JAW.—See Tetanus.

LŒMIA.—Plague.

LŒMOCHOLOSIS.—Yellow Fever.

LOOSENESS.—Diarrhœa.

LOW SPIRITS.—Hypochondriasis.

LUCOMANIA.—Lycanthropia.

LUES.—Disease, Plague, Syphilis.

LUMBAGO.—Rheumatism of the Lumbar Region, Stitch in the Back. A spasmodic affection of the muscles of the loins, attended with pain, and often inability to walk. Fomentations will relieve the pain, after which the paroxysms are to be prevented by restoring the general health.

LUMBAR ABSCESS.—Psoas Abscess. An apostema or abscess in the lumbar region. The suppuration is often profuse, and attended with severe and exhausting hectic. In the early stage, the inflamed part should be kept constantly covered with cold wet cloths very frequently renewed, and the whole surface bathed once or twice a day with tepid water, or, if the superficial temperature is considerable, the wet-sheet pack should be employed daily. The dietary must be exceedingly abstemious.

LUNATIC.—Moonstruck. One who has lost the use of his reasoning powers.

LUNATISMUS.—Somnambulism.

LUNG FEVER.—See Pneumonitis.

LUPUS.—Tubercular Ulcer. *Noli me Tangere.* Tubercular Excrescences about the nose, with ragged, spreading ulcerations. Sometimes they appear in the cheek where they destroy the part deeply. The disorganized mass should be at once destroyed with caustic.

LUXATION.—Dislocation; Displacement of a part from its normal position; putting out of joint.

LYCANTHE.—Hydrophobia, Dry Choak, Wolf Choak.

LYCANTHROPIA.—A variety of melanholy in which the person believes himself changed into a wolf.

LYMPHADENITIS.—Inflammation of a gland.

LYSSA.—Hydrophobia.

MACIES.—Atrophy, Emaciation.

MACULA.—A spot. Permanent Discoloration of the Skin.

MAD.—Insane.

MADAROSIS.—Loss of the Hair. Depilitation.

MADNESS, CANINE.—Hydrophobia.

MADOR.—A cold sweat. A symptom in low fevers, and various conditions of exhaustion.

MAGGOT PIMPLE.—See Acne.

MAL DES ARDENS.—A malignant Erysipelas which prevailed epidemically in France in 1130.

MAL DE CRIMEE.—A kind of Leprosy in the Crimea.

MAL DEL SOLE.—Pellagra.

MALACIA.—Depravation of taste. General loathing of food with an exclusive longing for some particular article. It affects some pregnant women, and is a symptom in several nervous and dyspeptic affections. Whether the appetite should be restrained or indulged, depends entirely on the nature of the article craved.

MALADY.—Disease, Sickness.

MALADY, ENGLISH.—Hypochondriasis.

MALAISE.—Indisposition.

MALARIA.—Miasm.

MALASSIMILATION.—Imperfect or Morbid Nutrition.

MALIGNANT.—Applied to any very dangerous disease.

MALVERNMANIA.—I introduce this *mad* technicality for the purpose of quoting an instructive paragraph from DUNGLISON's Medical Dictionary, page 565:

"MALVERN, WATERS OF.—The village of Great Malvern, (pronounced *Maw*-vern,) in Worcestershire, England, has for many years been celebrated for a spring of remarkable purity, which has acquired the name of the *Holy well*. It is a carbonated water, containing carbonates of soda and iron, sulphate of soda, and chloride of sodium; and is chiefly used externally in cutaneous affections."

How can water be "remarkably pure" when it is strongly impregnated with half-a-dozen impurities surpasses my comprehension altogether. Nor is the puzzle at all unpuzzled when the same author informs us on page 912 that, water is composed of eight parts by weight of oxygen, and one of hydrogen. If pure water consists of oxygen and hydrogen, how much *purer* does the addition or admixture of such drugs as soda, iron, sulphur, and salt, make it?

MAMAPIAN.—A malignant erosive ulcer.

MAMMARY ABSCESS.—Mastodynia Apostematosa, Mastitis.

Milk Abscess.—Phlegmonous inflammation of the heart, usually incident to the lying-in period. It requires cold local applications in the outset, with tepid ablutions for the general feverishness. Should the disease progress to suppuration, indicated by a sense of extreme tension and throbbing pain, a bread-and-milk or elm flour poultice should be applied; and when pus has actually formed, the abscess should be opened with a lancet.

MANGE.—Itch of Animals. A cutaneous disease to which all domesticated animals are liable, and which especially affects the horse, cow, sheep, and dog. Uncleanliness is the obvious cause, and I need hardly add that cleanliness is the remedy. Too many of our farmers allow their animals to stand over and sleep on their own accumulated excrement, which poisons them all through, and sickens or vitiates those who eat their flesh, drink their milk, or inhale their breath, to say nothing of typhoid fevers, malignant erysipelas, putrid sore throat, diptheria, and contagious diseases generally, which their owners and neighbors are liable to from such filthy associations.

MANIA.—Terror, Madness, Insanity, Delirium. The term is commonly restricted to *furious* or *raving insanity.* DUNGLISON says "Mania attacks adults chiefly; and women more frequently than men." Such expressions exhibit in a striking light the absurd notions which are entertained of the nature of diseases. Maladies of all kinds, mental as well as bodily, are regarded and treated as *entities;* as something extraneous to the living organism, and acting upon it, or as the phrase is *"attacking"* it. When this false dogma—this *mania* of the medical profession is exploded, and disease is understood to be *the action of the living system itself*, there will be a revolution in medical science, and a reform in the healing art. Many cases of mania are immediately caused by constipation, bad blood, and their consequences, congestion of, or "rush of blood" to the brain, and are curable by the appropriate hygienic appliances. When dependant on dissipation, nervous exhaustion, or organic lesions, the asylum is the proper place for the patient.

MANIA, DANCING.—Dancing Plague, St. John's Dance, Tarantism, St. Vitus's Dance. A convulsive malady, which prevailed epidemically, in various parts of Europe during the middle ages, and more or less connected with religious excitements. Similar affections have been manifested in various parts of the United States. When one or more persons are exercised in this manner, the malady is easily propagated sympathetically. Proper restraint, and a sufficiency of the "Hunger-Cure," will prove infallible as remedies.

MANIA, EPILEPTIC.—Epilepsy.

MANIA A POTU.—Delirium Tremens.

MANIA, PUERPERAL.—Insanity during childbed.

MARASMUS.—Atrophy, Emaciation. Wasting of the body without fever or inflammation. It is really a form of indigestion. The term is usually applied to dyspeptic infants or children.

MARASMUS SENILIS.—Atrophy of the aged.

MARASMUS TABES.—Tabes Dorsalis. Atrophy from sexual abuse.

MASTITIS.—Inflammation of the Breast. See Mammary Abscess.

MASTODYNIA.—Mastalgia. Neuralgia of the Breast. The term is sometimes applied also to Mammary Abscess.

MASTONCUS.—A Tumor of the Breast or Nipple.

MASTORRHAGIA.—Excessive Flow of Milk. Cold applications and a dry diet are the remedies.

MASTURBATION.—Self Pollution; Onanism.

MATERIA MEDICA.—A term applied to the sum total of the materials employed as medicines. I predict that before many years have elapsed, the phrase, Materia *Morbus*, will be substituted.

MATURATION.—Progression of an abscess to suppuration.

MEASLES.—See Rubeola.

MEGRIM.—Hemicrania.

MELÆNE.—Black Jaundice. A term applied to the vomiting and purging of black matter. It is also sometimes applied to hemorrhage from the bowels.

MELANCHOLY.—Lypemania, Ecphronia. Mental alienation characterized by mistrust, depression, and gloom. Thick blood, torpid liver, constipated bowels, nervous exhaustion, etc., are the common causes. Prolonged religious or other mental excitement, and intense mental occupation, are predisposing causes.

MELANCHOLY, EROTIC.—Erotomania. Melancholy or monomania occasioned by restrained sexual passion.

MELANOSIS.—Black Tubercle, Black Cancer, Fungus Melanodes. Conversion of the tissue into a black, hard, homogeneous substance, near which cavities and ulcers form. This morbific change is owing to the deposit of tuberculous matter; and the deposit is owing to retained effete and unassimilable chylous or nutrient matter. It is met with in the lungs, liver, areolar tissue, and other parts. It is to be treated as a cachexy, and this means that all possible processes of purification and invigoration should be resorted to.

MELASMA.—See Ecchymoma.

MELICERIS.—An encysted tumor filled with a substance of the consistency of honey. It requires excision.

MELITIS.—Inflammation of the Cheek.

MELOÆMIA.—Putrescent state of the Blood.

MEMBRANE, FALSE.—The concreted fibrinous excretion which exudes on membraneous surfaces, as in Croup, Diptheria, Dysmenorrhœa, Catarrh of the Bladder, Tubercular Diarrhœa, etc. A similar exudation sometimes takes place on ulcerated surfaces.

MENINGITIS.—Meningiitis. Inflammation of the meninges or membranes, usually applied to those of the brain and spinal cord. The distinction which authors make between inflammation of the substance or parenchyma of an organ, and its investing coat or membrane, is neither useful nor practical. Both are more or less involved in the disease, and the treatment is precisely the same whether one or both are affected, or in whatever degree they are relatively disordered.

MENINGO-CEPHALITIS.—Inflammation of the brain and its membranes. See Cephalitis.

MENORRHAGIA.—Excessive loss of blood at the menstrual periods. The term is often employed synonymously with uterine hemorrhage. Its essential causes are laxity and obstruction. The hemorrhage should be arrested by means of quiet in the horizontal posture, cold cloths to the abdomen, and cold vaginal injections. In severe cases ice should be introduced into the vagina, or cold water introduced into the rectum. If these measures do not restrain the bleeding, the introduction of a soft sponge to the os uteri is necessary. The apartment of the patient should be well ventilated, but the temperature should be comfortable. Care must be taken to keep the extremities warm. The recurrence of the hemorrhage can only be prevented by restoring the tone and vigor of the whole muscular system.

MENOSTASIA.—See Amenorrhœa.

MENSES ALBA.—Leucorrhœa.

MENSIUM RETÉNTIO.—Retention of the Menstrual Flux. See Amenorrhœa.

MENSTRUATION DIFFICILE.—Dysmenorrhœa.

9

MENSTRUATION VICARIOUS.—Paramenia Erroris. Hemorrhage from other than the reproductive organs, at the time of menstruation. It is to be cured by restoring the normal menstruation.

MENTAGRA.—Sycosis.

MEPHITIC.—Unwholesome Exhalations.

MERCURIAL HUMOR.—A term anciently applied to a supposititious humor which occasions melancholy.

MERCURIALISMUS.—Hydrargyriasis. Mercurial Disease.

MERCURIALIZATION.—The Poisoning by Mercury, Mercurial Fever, Mercurial Cachexy.

MEROCELE.—Mirocele. Femoral or Crural Hernia.

MEROCOXALGIA.—See Coxalgia.

MEROPIA.—Partial Obscurity of Vision.

MERORRHEUMA.—Tropical Rheumatism.

MESENTERITIS.—Inflammation of the Mesentery. The symptoms are similar to those of *Peritonitis*, (of which it is a variety,) but milder and more obscure. The treatment is the same, though less in degree. See Peritonitis.

MESMERIZATION.—A state of Mental Passivity or of Insensibility, induced by what is vaguely termed "animal magnetism."

MESMERIZATION.—Magnetization. The state of being mesmerized, or the act of magnetizing.

MESMERIZED.—An abnormal condition induced by the process or influence called *animal* magnetism, in which the patient is insensible, or acts according to the volition of the operator. The sleep induced by magnetism is termed *Hypnotization*.

METADERMATOSIS.—Morbid development of the epidermis.

METALLODYNIA.—Pain caused by minerals, as lead, quicksilver, etc.

METAMORPHOPSIA.—Phantasmatoscopia, False Sight. An affection of the eyes in which the patient recognizes objects which are merely imaginary. The objects may be cob-webs, insects, pieces of wood, black spots, etc., and are perpetually moving. They are sometimes called *Maculæ Volitantes*. They may be owing to over-exertion of the eyes, or to thickening or deposits in the coats or humors. Rest of the organs and purification of the blood are the measures to arrest the difficulty and prevent total loss of vision.

METAPTOSIS.—Change in the form or seat of a disease.

METASTASIS.—Morbid Translation; Change in the seat of a disease. The prevailing medical theories of metastatic disease are both absurd and amusing. Gout and rheumatism often "change" from one joint or place to another; cutaneous affections on being "cured" on the surface appear, or as the saying is, "re-appear" on the mucous surface of the alimentary canal, or in the membranes of the brain; mumps when "scattered" from the neck affect the testes or breasts; measles when "repelled" from the skin "locate" on the pulmonary mucous membrane; morbid humors when "discussed" from the outside "attack" the inside, etc. The Humoral Pathologists attributed the "phenomena" to a "translation" of the morbific matter to a new locality or different part; and the Solidists, to the transfer or displacement of the "irritation." There is no unmuddling this muddlement on any of the theories of disease except that of the Hygeio-Therapeutic school, which regards disease as remedial action. When the remedial effort is checked or prevented in one place or direction, it becomes more manifest, active, and apparent in another, just as the action of the kidneys are increased by diminishing the action of the skin, and *vice versa*. This principle shows at a glance the vast importance of the universal rule in medicating all diseases—balancing the circulation and thereby equalizing the remedial effort; and it shows also the rationale of the dangerous and often fatal results of "curing one disease by producing another," or, in other words, *of poisoning* a person because he is sick. Metastatic affections require precisely the same treatment as do the same diseases when idiopathic.

METHOMANIA.—Irresistible Desire for Intoxicating Substances, **Temulentia.**   A madness or depravity of the instincts caused by the use of stimulants.   All of the morbid appetences, with their consequences, gluttony, drunkenness, dissipation, debauchery, and sensuality, may be traced to stimulation as the parent or primary cause.

METRALGIA.—Pain in the Uterus.

METRITIS.—Hysteritis, Inflammation of the Womb.   The symptoms are, pain, swelling, and tenderness in the lower part of the abdomen, with heat and tenderness of the os uteri.   Vomiting is usually an accompaniment, and there is fever of either the entonic or atonic diathesis—commonly the latter.

Cold applications to the part, tepid or cool vaginal injections, tepid hip-baths, and tepid ablutions are the proper bathing processes.   In very low states of the system, the full warm bath, and fomentations to the abdomen are preferable.

METROCARCINOMA.—Cancer of the Uterus.

METRODYNIA.—Metralgia.

METROMANIA.—See Nymphomanja.

METROPERITONITIS.—Puerperal Fever.   See Peritonitis.

METROPROPTOSIS.—Prolapsus Uteri.

METRORRHAGIA.—Uterine Hemorrhage.   Bleeding from the uterus, at the menstrual period or at other times, but in excessive quantity.   When it occurs after delivery it requires to be promptly arrested or death may speedily result.   Indeed, hemorrhage is one of the most dreaded complications of the young *accoucheur*.   The remedial measures are, the horizontal posture, cold wet cloths to the abdomen, thighs and loins, injections of the coldest water into the vagina, and, in extreme cases, plugging the vagina with soft cloths or lint, so as to induce a coagulation and close the bleeding vessels.   The patient should have an abundance of fresh, cool air.

MIASMA.—Deleterious affluvia arising from decaying or decomposing organic matter.   *Marsh miasma*—malaria—which arise from rotting vegetation, are among the chief causes of intermittent fevers.

MILIARY FEVER.—Miliaria, Sudatoria, Millet-seed Rash. One of the exanthems or eruptive fevers; so called from the small, red, numerous, and slightly raised pimples which appear on the surface. In about twenty-four hours the pimples become vesicles, filled with a whitish and transparent fluid. The fever is continued in type and atonic in diathesis, and is accompanied with a sour sweat, which is often profuse. It is caused by too much external heat, confined air, slop food, hot drinks, irritating condiments, etc. Women in the puerperal state, when improperly nursed, are quite subject to it. The treatment is very simple—quiet, and tepid ablutions.

MILK ABSCESS.—See Mammary Abscess.

MILK FEVER.—See Fever, Milk.

MILK LEG.—Phlegmasia Dolens, White Leg, Swelled Leg, White Swelling of Lying-in Women. An inflammatory affection, commonly limited to one leg, which occurs a few days after delivery. It is hot, white, unyielding, and gives to the touch a sensation of numerous irregular prominences under the skin. It is attended with considerable feverishness; the pressure of the gravid uterus, in a plethoric state of the system, interrupting the circulation of the neighboring veins and absorbents, and inducing serous effusion into the areolar tissue, is probably the rationale of the malady. Cold wet cloths, frequently renewed, until the morbid heat subsides, tepid ablutions whenever the external temperature calls for them, and due attention to the bowels, comprise the remedial plan.

MILK SCALL.—Porrigo Larvalis.

MILK-SICKNESS.—Swamp-Sickness, Sick Stomach, Trembles, Slows, Tires, Stiff-joints, River-Sickness, Puking Fever. A form of putrid typhus fever which has occurred in some parts of Alabama, Indiana, Kentucky, and the other Western States, characterized by excruciating pain in the knee and other joints, with general tremors. It affects cows and other animals in certain seasons, and those persons who feed on their flesh or drink their milk, and is undoubtedly caused by poisonous or rotting vegetation which the animals take with their food. It is generally endemic ; another fact which points to the origin above indicated.   The malady is commonly attended with vomiting and purging, and extreme nervous agitation.   The patient should take frequent sips of cold or iced-water ; cold wet cloths should be applied over the stomach and abdomen, well covered with dry flannel, and frequently changed ; the whole surface sponged with tepid water two or three times a day, and the extremities kept warm with hot bottles.

MILLET-SEED RASH.—Miliary Fever.

MISANTHROPIA.—Misanthropy ; aversion to man and to society.   It is a symptom of melancholy, hypochondriasis, and various other forms of indigestion.

MISCARRIAGE.—Abortion.

MOANING.—Plaintive and Audible Respiration.   A sign of great oppression or congestion in some internal organ.

MOGIGRAPHIA.—Writers' Cramp.   Spasmodic rigidity of some of the muscles of the fingers and arms, in consequence of close application with the pen or pencil.

MOLE.—A fleshy, insensible mass, soft or hard, of variable size, which sometimes forms in the uterus.   It has been supposed to be the result of impregnation with imperfect development, and hence called *False* Conception ; but moles are occasionally found in the virgin uterus.   The diseased mass may or may not contain parts of a fetus.   It is expelled as in cases of abortion, and requires the same management.

MOLLITIES.—Preternatural softening of an organ or texture.

MOLLITIES, CEREBRI.—Encephalomalacia ; Softening of the Brain ; Mollescence or liquefaction of some portion of the cerebral substance.   This condition is never certainly known till revealed by a post-mortem examination, and it exists in the imaginations of physicians and patients a hundred times as often as it exists in the brains of the latter.   Various strange and indescribable sensations which affect the heads and disturb the mental operations of dyspeptic and nervous invalids, especially those who have long suffered of constipated bowels, are often vaguely referred to a supposed *softening of the brain*. *Hardening of the bowels* is nearer the truth. To relieve the head medicate the bowels.

MOLLITIES CORDIS.—Cardiomalacia.

MOLLITIES MEDULLÆ SPINALIS.—Ramollissement; Softening of the Spinal Marrow. An affection often suspected, but seldom known to exist. When it does exist it is incurable.

MOLLITIES OSSIUM.—Softening of the Bones. A rare affection, and owing to defective assimilation; in other words, a remote effect of indigestion. The disease generally affects the whole bony structure, and the urine contains large portions of phosphate of lime. Medical authors do not pretend that it is ever curable, and it is clear that no remedial measures can avail, except such as tend to restore the primary nutritive functions.

MOLLUSCUM.—Atheroma. Numerous tumors varying in size from that of a pea to that of a pigeon's egg, or even larger, filled with a fatty or pulpy matter, developed in the substance of the skin, are so called from their resemblance to certain molluscuous animals. Cleanliness, a simple and abstemious diet, with frequent ablutions and gentle friction, are the remedies.

MOLOPES.—Vibices.

MOLYBDOSIS.—Lead-Poisoning.

MONOBLEPSIS.—Confused vision only when both eyes are employed.

MONOMANIA.—Mania or derangement of one of the mental powers; madness or hallucination in relation to some particular person, object, or theme

MONOPATHY.—Disease of a single mental organ.

MORBI, MORBUS.—See Disease.

MORPHEW.—Scurfy Eruptions of the Face.

MORPION.—Crab Louse. See Pediculus.

MORTIFICATION.—Loss of Vitality in a part of the Body.

The incipient stage is called *Gangrene;* total death is called *Sphacelus.* Mortification of bone is called *Necrosis.*

MOTHER'S MARKS.—Spots. See Nævus.

MULLIGRUBS.—Tormina, Colic.

MUMPS.—See Parotis.

MUR.—Coryza.

MURR.—Pestilential Fever; Murrain. An epizootic disease, commonly regarded as contagious, having some resemblance to small-pox, which affects cattle, especially sheep. It is said to have been transferred to man. The treatment is the same as for small-pox. See Variola.

MUSICOMANIA, MUSOMANIA.—Monomania for Music. The passion for music so strong as to derange the intellect.

MUSSITATIO.—A motion of the tongue and lips, as in the act of speaking, but without any sound. It is a bad symptom, and indicates great oppression of the brain or lungs.

MUTITAS.—Dumbness, Speechlessness.

MUTITAS SUDORUM.—Deaf-dumbness.

MYALGIA.—Cramp, which see.

MYELITIS.—Inflammation of the spinal marrow or its membranes. It is characterized by deep-seated, burning pain in the spine, with general feverishness, and a variety of distressing sensations usually called "nervous." It is a rare disease, and much oftener suspected than proved to exist.

MYOPIA, MYOPY.—Purblindness, Mouse-sight, Shortsightedness. It may be palliated by wearing concave glasses.

MYOSIS.—Permanent contraction of the pupil. It is usually a result of iritis.

MYOSITIS.—Myitis, Mysitis; Acute Rheumatism.

MYRINGITIS.—Inflammation of the Ear Drum.

NÆVUS.—Maculæ Matricis, Fancy Marks, Mother's Marks, Mother's Spots. Various spots on the skin with which children are born, are so designated. Some are very superficial—mere stains; others are prominent; while some are largely composed of anastomosing blood-vessels. The latter only are properly medicable, and may generally be removed by proper surgery.

NARCOSIS.—Stupor, Stupefaction.. The state of torpor and insensibility occasioned by narcotic drugs, as opium, henbane, belladonna, etc. The usual practice of exciting, stimulating, exercising, and galvanizing narcotized patients only makes a bad matter worse. The patient should have profound quiet, abundance of fresh air, cold applications to the head and warm to the feet. When there is reason to suspect the presence of the drug in the stomach, the stomach, or a warm water emetic should be employed.

NAUSEA.—Squeasiness, Sickness, Inclination to Vomit. Symptomatic of many diseases and morbid conditions. Warm water-drinking until whatever offensive material may exist in the stomach is removed, then sips of iced-water, or bits of ice to swallow, with cold wet cloths to the epigastrium, are the general remedies.

NAUSEA, KREATIC.—The sickness and vomiting which animal food, in any quantity however small, occasions in some persons. Vegetarianism is an infallible preventive!

NAUSEA, MARINA.—Sea-Sickness. A very abstemious and simple dietary will usually prevent and always mitigate this distressing affection. Wearing a rather tight girdle around the region of the epigastrium will lessen and often remove it. The horizontal posture will also relieve the paroxysm more or less, and often prevent it altogether. Many persons will become sick in the ship's cabin, when the sea is rough, who are entirely free of it, so long as they are on deck. If our ship-builders would properly ventilate the cabins and berths—and it is not difficult nor expensive to do so—they would save the passengers an immense amount of suffering.

NEAR-SIGHTEDNESS.—Myopia.

NEBULA.—Nubes, Nephelion. A slight speck on the cornea. It is also applied to a mist or cloud suspended in the urine. See Caligo.

NECK, DERBYSHIRE.—See Bronchocele.

NECROPHOBIA.—Exaggerated Fear of Death. A common
9*

symptom in hypochondriasis. It is regarded as a bad symptom when occurring in fevers.

NECROPNEUMONIA.—Gangrene of the Lungs. It occurs in bad cases of putrid pneumonitis, and is indicated by extreme fetor of the breath and expectoration. When circumscribed it is not necessarily fatal.

NEPHRALGIA.—Pain or Neuralgia in the Kidney.

NEPHRITIS.—Inflammation of the Kidney. The symptoms are, acute pain, burning heat and sense of weight, suppression or diminution of urine, retraction of the testicle, and numbness of the thigh of the affected side, and fever. Cool hip-baths, tepid ablutions, and, when the fever is of the entonic diathesis, the wet-sheet pack, are the leading measures of treatment.

NEPHRITIS ALBUMENSIS.—BRIGHT'S Disease of the Kidney.

NEPHROLITHIASIS.—See Gravel.

NEPHROMALACIA.—Softening of the Kidney.

NEPHRORRHAGIA.—Hæmaturia Renalis; Hemorrhage of the Kidney. See Hæmaturia.

NERVINE.—The term is defined to be, "a medicine which acts on the nervous system." A proper definition is, abnormal vital action, with a more especial disturbance of the normal functions of the nervous tissue. Instead of the medicine acting on the nervous system, the reverse is true.

NERVOUS.—The term is employed *physiologically* in the sense of active, vigorous, strong; and *pathologically* in the sense of weak, irritable, and frail.

NERVOUSNESS.—Nervous Diathesis, Abnormal sensibility, or preternatural irritability. A vague term.

NERVOUS DISEASES.—Diseases whose symptoms are most prominently manifested by the nervous system.

NERVOUS PAIN.—Neuralgia.

NEURALGIA.—Neurodynia, Tic Douloureux, Nerve Pain. A disease characterized by acute, darting pain along the course of a nerve, without fever. It is always symptomatic of obstruction, exhaustion, or the effects of mineral or narcotic drugs. Very hot applications will sometimes give relief, and in other cases very cold are best; while in still others, alternate warm and cold applications are preferable.

NEURITIS.—Inflammation of a Nerve; Neuralgia.

NEURODYNIA.—Neuralgia.

NEUROMA.—Subcutaneous and highly painful tumors formed on the tissue of the nerves.

NEUROMALACIA.—Softening of the Nerves.

NEVUS.—See Nævus.

NICTATION.—Twinkling of the Eye. It sometimes becomes a morbid habit, to be overcome by "moral suasion."

NOCTAMBULISMUS.—Somnambulism.

NOCTURNAL EMISSIONS.—See Spermatorrhœa.

NODDLE-POX.—Syphilimania.

NODE.—Nodus. A hard concretion or incrustation which forms around gouty and rheumatic joints. They are often occasioned by mercurial medicines.

NOLI ME TANGERE.—See Lupus.

NOSE-BLEED.—See Epistaxis.

NOSE, RUNNING AT THE.—See Coryza.

Nosos.—Disease.

NOSTALGIA.—Nostomania, Home-Sickness. Emaciation of the body, commonly attended with hectic, occasioned by the desire of returning to one's home or country. It is a species of melancholy.

NURSING SORE MOUTH.—See Apthæ.

NYCLATOPIA.—See Hemeralopia.

NYMPHITIS.—Inflammation of the Clitoris.

NYMPHOMANIA.—Furor Uterinus, Uteromania. Insatiable desire in females for sexual commerce. Its immediate cause is an inflammatory condition of the sexual organs; its remote

causes are, constipation, irritating condiments, gross food, masturbation, obscene literature, etc.

The prolonged tepid bath, with frequent hip-baths of a moderate temperature, and a plain, abstemious dietary, are the remedies. The patient sometimes becomes perfectly maniacal, when solitude is indispensable.

OARITIS.—Inflammation of the Ovarium. The *acute* form is rare. In *chronic* oarities the symptoms are very obscure. The chief ones are pain, heat, and sense of weight in the lower part of the abdomen, aggravated at the menstrual periods. These symptoms also attend the incipient stage of *Ovarian Tumor*, but in this case there is gradually progressing enlargement noticeable externally. Hip-baths, the wet girdle, and a rigidly simple dietary are the specialities.

OBESITY. — Polysarcia, Corpulency, Fatness, Morbid accumulation of adipose matter in the system. It means excessive alimentation with defective depuration, and its causes are, too much or too gross food, or deficient exercise, or both. Correct these habits and the surplus fat will be duly eliminated. I have had patients who had accumulated one, two, and in one case, nearly three hundred pounds of this effete matter. Such persons are liable to die at any moment of "apoplexy," or congestion in some vital part.

OBSTIPATIO.—Constipation.

OCCLUSION.—Imperforation, as of the vagina, pupil, etc.

ODONTAGRA.—Dentagra. Arthritic pain in the Teeth.

ODONTALGIA.—Toothache. It is generally caused by inflammation, and is usually connected with caries, which exposes the cavity to the contact of air, and other extraneous matters. Fasting, warm hip-baths, hot and cold foot-baths, cold applications to the head, and tepid or cool water held in the mouth, are the remedial resources.

ODONTITIS.—Inflammation of the Teeth. See Odontalgia.

ODONTOLITHOS. — Tartar; Incrustation of the Teeth. It consists of phosphate of lime, mucus, some animal substance, and a small quantity of salivary matter. Infusoria have been found in these incrustations. The tooth-brush, or rinsing in the morning, and after meals, will be sufficient, if the secretions of the mouth are normal, and the diet proper. A *very* stiff brush should not be used, as it might injure the enamel. When the tartar accumulates in spite of this measure, it should be removed by the dentist.

ODONTOSTERESIS.—Loss of the Teeth. Hot drinks, slop-food, condiments, especially salt and vinegar, and alkaline and mineral drugs, are the usual causes of the prevalent rotting out of the teeth. It is as unnatural and unnecessary for the teeth to decay prematurely, as it is for the eyes, or ears, or fingers, or toes, to do so. Very few teeth would ever decay if all the food taken was properly masticated.

ŒDEMA.—Hydrops Cellularis. Accumulation of serous fluid in the areolar tissue. The swelling is soft, pits on pressure, and preserves the indentation for some time. See Anasarca.

ŒDEMA ARSENICALIS.—Swelling of the face and eyelids from the prolonged use of arsenic.

ŒDEMA OF THE GLOTTIS.—Œdematous Laryngitis, Hydro-pneumonia. An inflammatory affection with serous or sero-purulent infiltration into the submucous tissue of the glottis. The symptoms very much resemble those of croup, but has less fever and cough, with more difficulty of breathing in the early stages. It also commonly affects adults, whereas croup usually affects children. The prompt and persevering application of cold wet cloths externally, and ice or iced-water internally, are the main remedial resources. Of course, due attention should be paid to the state of the bowels, and the general feverishness.

ŒDEMA LACTEUM.—Phlegmatia Dolens. See Milk Leg.

ŒDEMA OF THE LUNGS.—Hydrops Pulmonum, Hydro-pneumonia, Infiltration of serum into the Lungs. It is one of the effects of maltreated pneumonia. The cough is attended with aqueous expectoration, and the respiration is laborious.

Bleeding and antimony are the most frequent causes of this condition of the lungs.

Œsophagismus.—Dysphasia Spasmodica, Stricture of the Œsophagus. It may be spasmodic, or a thickening of the mucous membrane; in either case the dietary is the essential thing to manage in the treatment. Salt, grease, milk, and sugar are especially to be avoided.

Œsophagitis.—Inflammatory Dysphagia; Inflammation of the Œsophagus.

Omentitis.—Inflammation of the Omentum. See Peritonitis.

Omphalorrhagia. — Unlimited Hemorrhage. New-born infants are liable to it. Cold water or ice will arrest it.

Onanism.—Self-Abuse, Masturbation.

Oneirodynia.—Painful Dreams; Incubus and Somnambulism are examples.

Onychia.—Paronychia.

Onychitis.—Inflammation of a Nail.

Onychonosi.—Disease of the Nails.

Onychoptosis.—Falling of the Nails.

Onyx.—Pterygion. A collection of purulent matter between the laminæ of the cornea, having the shape of a nail. It is a proper subject for surgery.

Opacity.—In pathology, applied to a fluid or structure which has lost its transparency, or the cornea or crystalline lens of the eyes.

Opisthotonos.—Tetanus with inclination backward. See Tetanus.

Ophthalmia. — Ophthalmitis; Inflammation of the Eye. The various forms of this disease have received numerous appellations, as they involve more or less the different structures of the eye and its appendages. These will be treated of under their respective names. The three leading forms, each of which has several varieties, are the *Membraneous* or *Conjunctival*, the *Egyptian* or *Purulent*, and the *Tarsal*. The fever attending Opthalmia may be of the entonic or atonic diathesis, while the inflammation is correspondingly phlegmonous or erysipelatous. In the treatment the room should be so darkened or shaded that the light will not be painful; wet or cold applications—always preferring the temperature that is most agreeable—should be constantly applied to the eyes; hip and foot baths are useful as derivatives; and the surface must be "packed" or sponged according to the diathesis of the fever. The bowels must be kept free with tepid enemas, and no food must be taken until the violence of the fever has subsided. Caustics and astringents should never be applied to inflamed eyes until the blood is well purified, and the heat and tenderness of the organs entirely abated. Thousands of eyes are destroyed because of inattention to this rule.

OPTHALMITIS.—See Opthalmia.

ORCHEITIS.—Inflammation of the Scrotum; Hernia Humoralis.

ORCHIOCELE.—Scrotal Hernia.

ORCHITIS.—Orcheitis.

ORTHOPNŒA.—Suffocation, Strangulation. Difficult breathing, especially in the horizontal posture.

ORTHOPNŒA, CARDIACA.—Angina Pectoris.

OSCHOCARCINOMA.—Chimney Sweepers' Cancer; Cancer of the Scrotum.

OSCHEOCELE.—See Hydrocele.

OSTALGITIS, OSTEITIS.—Inflammation of Bone.

OSTEMPYESIS.—An Abscess in the Interior of a Bone.

OSTEOCELE.—Induration of the Testicles.

OSTEOMA.—Exostosis.

OSTEOMALACIA, OSTEOMALACOSIS.—Mollities Ossium.

OSTEOPOROSIS.—Induration of Bone.

OSTEO-SARCOMA.—Cancerous Degeneration of Bone.

OSTEO-STEATOMA.—Bony Tumor.

OSTITIS.—Ostalgitis.

OSTOMA.—Exostosis.

OTAGRA, OTALGIA.—Pain in the Ear.

OTIRRHŒA.—Discharge of pus from the ear ; a symptom of chronic otitis.

OTITIS.—Inflammation of the Ear. When acute the symptoms are, excruciating pain, with intolerable burning, and a discharge of mucus' from the external meatus, or from the Eustachian tube. The treatment is substantially the same as for Opthalmia.

OTOPYORRHŒA.—Otirrhœa.

OVARIAN TUMOR.—Hydrops Ovarii ; Encysted Dropsy of the Ovary. It may be distinguished from *Ascites* by the enlargement commencing at one side of the lower portion of the abdomen, and gradually extending upward and over the whole abdomen. The early stage is accompanied with more or less menstrual disturbance, often noticeable only each alternate month—a fact which strikingly corroborates the theory that ovulation is alternate with the right and left ovaries, and that the law of sex is thereby to be determined.* In the later stages of ovarian dropsy the treatment can only be palliative. In the early stages I have succeeded in arresting the disease in several cases. The dietary must be rigidly abstemious, and the wet-sheet applied daily for an hour, if the strength and temperature of the patient will permit. Local applications are of little consequence, unless there is mismenstruation in some form, in which case the treatment must be regulated accordingly. Extirpation of the diseased mass has been practiced with success in many cases, but a majority operated upon have not recovered. Paracentesis will give temporary relief; but as the fluid is accumulated in several sacs, but a small portion of it can be removed.

OVARITIS.—Oaritis.

OXYOPIA.—Inordinate Acuteness of the Sense of Sight.

OXYOSPHRESIA.—Inordinate Acuteness of the Sense of Smell.

---

* This subject will be fully discussed in the Author's forthcoming work, "Sexual Physiology Complete."

OXYPHLEGMASIA.—Violent Inflammation.

OZÆNA.—Malignant Coryza. An affection of the mucous membrane of the nose and throat, owing to caries of the bones, or connected with syphilitic or mercurial infection, and attended with a disagreeable odor like that of a crushed bed-bug. The remedy is purification of the whole system.

PACHÆMIA.—Morbid Thickness of the Blood. Inactivity of the liver, and the excessive use of grease, sugar, and other hydro-carbonaceous articles of diet, are the common causes. Constipated bowels indirectly conduce to the same result; hence persons who are habitually costive are constantly liable to congestion of the brain and lungs, palpitation, piles, and other manifestations of a disordered circulation.

PACHEABLEPHAROSIS.—Thickening of the eyelids from tubercles or excrescences formed on their margins.

PAIN.—Morbid Sensation. It denotes the presence of some morbific agent, or some abnormal condition; its rationale is, doubtless, distention of the blood-vessels or contraction of the muscular fibers, so that the nerves are compressed. When the pressure is so great as to interrupt the transmission of nervous influence, there is loss of feeling, as in palsy, apoplexy, etc. There are many kinds of pain, as acute, dull, burning, itching, lancinating, griping, constant, remittent, lacerating, forcing, gnawing, grinding, etc., each of which is important in diagnosis. The practice of "curing" pain by means of opiates, narcotics, bleeding, etc., is founded on an erroneous theory of the nature of disease. Opium is more extensively employed in medicine than any other drug, because it is the most convenient agent to allay pain. But it does this by silencing the outcries of nature. The vital instincts proclaim that there is an enemy within the vital domain, and, in the language of *pain*, they call for help—for such materials and influences as they can use in expelling the morbific cause, and in repairing the damages. The doctor poisons them with a drug, which is resisted with such intensity in another direction as to suppress the original effort—and this he calls a *cure!*

The whole process resolves into curing the disease by killing the patient. Hygienic agencies relieve pain by supplying the conditions which nature requires to overcome or expel its cause.

PAINS, AFTER.—The pains which succeed delivery. They are occasioned by coagula, or retained *secundæ*, which excite the expulsive action of the uterus.

PAINS, LABOR.—Pains of Parturition. They are caused by the contraction of the uterus and adjacent muscles in the act of expelling its contents, or in the preparations therefor. The excessive pain and agony which females suffer in childbirth are owing wholly to the morbid and inflammatory condition which results necessarily from the ordinary habits of living and drugging.

PALENESS.—Pallor, Leucosis, Whiteness of Complexion. It implies determination of blood *from* the surface, and congestion in the internal organs.

PALPITATION.—A term applied to the heart's action when the individual is more sensible of it than ordinarily. When the action is forcible, the pulsations are called *throbbing;* and when very frequent, *fluttering*. Palpitations are sometimes connected with organic disease of the heart, but much more frequently by nervous and dyspeptic conditions. The most prolific cause of all is constipation of the bowels. The remedial plan must be directed to the removal of the obstruction, whatever that may be.

PALSY.—See Paralysis.

PALSY, LEAD.—See Paralysis Venenata.

PALSY, METALLIC.—See Paralysis Venenata

PALSY, SHAKING.—See Paralysis Agitans.

PALSY, PAINTERS.—See Paralysis Venenata.

PAMPLEGIA.—General Palsy; Paralysis of the whole body.

PANCREATITIS.—Inflammation of the Pancreas. The symptoms are very obscure, and perhaps the disease is never recognized during life.

PANDEMIC.—An epidemic which attacks the whole population.

PANDICULATION.—Stretching. It is indicative of fatigue, and is an effort to restore the balance of circulation.

PANTOPHOBIA.—Hydrophobia.

PANZOOTIA.—Epidemic Disease of Cattle.

PAPULA.—A Pimple; Exormia.

PARABYSOMA.—Engorgement of an organ; an enlargement consequent on accumulated blood.

PARALYSIS.—Palsy, Paresis. Partial or complete loss of sensation or motion, or both. Paralysis of one half of the body, vertically or horizontally, is termed *Hemiplegia;* of the lower half, *Paraplegia;* and of particular muscles or sets of muscles, *Local.*

Hemiplegia is more particularly connected with or caused by torpidity of the liver. I have never known a case in which disease of the liver was not a precedent condition, and sudden engorgement or congestion of that organ an exciting or immediate cause. The treatment should contemplate the purification of the mass of blood of its retained biliary matters as rapidly as possible. When the system is feverish, and the patient has not been drugged much, nor suffered long of chronic disease, the wet-sheet pack repeated daily will prove the most efficient detergent. In other cases tepid ablutions, followed by gentle, yet persevering friction, are to be preferred. *Cold* water should never be applied to the surface, except when and where there is preternatural heat. The bowels must be carefully attended to, and free evacuations produced, if necessary by means of injections of tepid water. When there is sense of weight and oppression with heat in the region of the liver, cold wet cloths, covered with dry, should be applied. In diet, the patient should be abstemious, and mainly frugivorous.

Paraplegia, when not the result of injury or mechanical violence, is more especially connected with, and caused by constipation of the bowels; hence persons of sedentary habits, gluttons, and those who are subject to great mental excitements, while their dietary is very constipating, are commonly the subjects of this form of palsy. The dripping sheet, or spray bath, daily or semi-weekly, hip-baths once or twice a day, the wet girdle during the night in cold weather, and a part of each day in warm weather, with a plain, vegetable and fruit diet, are the remedies. The patient should abstain from milk, fine flour, puddings, and all greasy dishes or articles.

Local palsy is produced by some specific poison, and the treatment must be directed to a removal of the cause, and a restoration of the circulation and sensibility of the part by bathing, friction, etc.

PARALYSIS AGITANS.—Shaking Palsy, Tremor, Trembling Palsy. A perpetual spasmodic agitation of the muscles. It is indicative of great nervous exhaustion, and is caused by mineral and narcotic drugs, extreme constipation of the bowels, sexual dissipation, etc. Many cases are incurable; and all that can be done remedially will be found in living in obedience to organic law, with such attentions to the functions of the excretory organs as the symptoms may clearly indicate.

PARALYSIS, BELL's.—A term which has been applied to paralysis of the muscles of the face, in consequence of a lesion of the *portio dura*, the nerve which supplies these muscles.

PARALYSIS BERIBERIA.—Beriberi. See Barbiers.

PARALYSIS VENENATA.—Paralysis caused by poisons, as of lead, mercury, ergot, arsenic, etc.

PARAMENIA.—Disordered Menstruation.

PARAPHIMOSIS.—Strangulation of the Glans Penis. Cold applications may so contract the part as to relieve it; if not the remedy consists in dividing the "bridle" formed by the prepuce.

PARAPHIA.—See Paralysis.

PARASITE.—Plants or animals which attach themselves to

other plants or animals are called *parasites*. Thus the mistletoe, which attaches itself to the oak, is a parasitic plant, and the louse or acari, which attach themselves to human beings and domestic animals, are parasitic animals. They occasion irritation, inflammation, ulceration, and feverishness, which are then termed *parasitic diseases*. Morbid growths, as tubercles, cancer, etc., are sometimes termed parasitic.

PARENCHYMATITIS.—Inflammation of the substance of an organ.

PARESIS.—Paralysis.

PARISTHMITIS.—Cynanche.

PARONYCHIA.—Whitlow, Felon, Onychia. A Phlegmonous tumor of the fingers or toes. Freezing the part a few times, for ten or fifteen minutes at a time, with some frigorific mixture, in the incipient stage, will generally arrest the disease. When the tension and pain become very great, the inflamed part should be divided freely, even down to the bones, and wet applications, of any temperature which is most soothing, continued as long as any inflammation exists.

PAROPSIS.—Disordered Vision.

PAROTIS, PAROTITIS.—Cynanche Parotidæ, Mumps. Inflammation of the Parotid Gland. The symptoms are, a painful tumefaction, with more or less heat and redness under the ear. A peculiar symptom of this disease is the benumbing sensation, when acids are taken into the mouth. The malady is usually epidemic, and has been long regarded as contagious; this is, however, very doubtful. In some cases it is accompanied with, or followed by an inflammatory affection of the testes in males and the breasts in females. Suppuration or induration is an occasional sequel of the disease, but commonly the inflammation terminates in resolution. Cold applications to the part, a very strict regimen, an equable temperature, and a daily ablution, are all the treatment the case ordinarily requires. The metastatic affections are to be treated precisely as should idiopathic affections of the parts, attended with the same symptoms.

PAROXYSM.—The hot, cold and sweating stages of febrile diseases; applied also to periodical exacerbations of any disease.

PARULIS.—Gum-Boil. Small abscesses in the gums, commonly occasioned by carious teeth.

PARURIA.—Morbid Excretion or Discharge of Urine.

PASSIVE.—When properly employed in pathology, this term denotes *atonic diathesis* in febrile and inflammatory affections, in contradistinction to *active*, which applies to entonic diathesis. In all visceral inflammations, when the fever is *typhoid* the local affection is *passive*. Authors speak of *active* internal congestion, *entonic* plethora, etc.; but these misapplications of language result from false theories of the nature of disease. Active congestion is always *external*, and only exists in inflammatory fever. Congestions of internal organs are always passive. Much erroneous and much *fatal* medical treatment would be avoided, if physicians understood the rationale of type and diathesis. These subjects will be explained fully in the author's work, "Principles of Hygienic Medication," now nearly ready for the press.

PATHEMA.—Affection; Disease.

PATHOLOGY.—The Doctrine of Disease. Pathology has been correctly defined as *disordered physiology;* but when authors speak or write of the "physiology of disease" they commit a most egregious blunder. They might as well tell us of the "*physiological effects*" of poisons—as indeed they do.

PATHOMANIA.—Moral Insanity. DUNGLISON defines it, "a *morbid* perversion of the natural feelings, affections, inclinations, temper, habits, moral disposition, and natural impulses," etc. This is like the "morbid poisons" we read of in medical books.

PATHOS.—Disease.

PELLAGRA.—A wrinkled and scaly appearance of the skin, especially in the parts exposed to the air, accompanied with debility, imbecility, cramps and convulsions. This singular malady has been noticed particularly among the Milanese, and has been supposed to follow the introduction of Indian corn. The method of cooking the corn, and the alkalies, salt, grease, sugar, etc., with which it is mixed or eaten, may have something to do with it. Tepid ablutions, abundant friction, air-baths, exposure of the naked body to light, air, and even sunshine, with a plain, unseasoned and solid dietary which secures thorough mastication, constitute the materia medica in the case.

PELLIALGIA.—Neuralgia of the Foot.

PEMPHIGUS.—Pompholyx, Serous Exanthem, Vesicular Fever, Bladdery Fever. This disease is characterized by vesicles scattered over the body, transparent, filbert-sized, with a red, inflamed edge, but without surrounding blush or tumefaction; on breaking they are liable to ulcerate; the fluid is slightly colored or transparent. The accompanying fever is continued and typhoid. Frequent ablutions with tepid water, and due attention to the bowels, are all the medication the patient requires.

PERICARDITIS.—Inflammation of the Pericardium. It cannot and need not be distinguished from *Carditis*.

PERICHONDRITIS.—Inflammation of the Perichondrium.

PERIOSTITIS.—Inflammation of the Periosteum.

PERIOSTOSIS.—A Tumor developed on Bone.

PERIPNEUMONIA.—Pneumonia, Pneumonitis.

PERIPNEUMONIA BILIOSA.—Bilious Pneumonia; Inflammation of the lungs with copious excretion of acrid bile. The term is commonly applied to what is properly called *Putrid Typhus Pneumonitis*; that is, pneumonitis, with typhus fever of the putrid form.

PERIPNEUMONIA CATARRHALIS.—This term has been indiscriminately applied to *Bronchitis, Influenza*, and *Peripneumonia Notha*.

PERIPNEUMONIA NOTHA.—Spurious Pneumonia, Bastard Pneumonia, Pseudo-Pneumonitis, False Pneumonia. These terms, with others as vague and erroneous, have been applied to that variety of Typhoid Pneumonia in which the fever is of the *nervous* form. Medical books are all in confusion on this subject, simply because they recognize either the local inflammation, or the general fever, to be primary or idiopathic, and the other secondary or symptomatic, instead of equal and essential parts of one and the same disease. See Pneumonitis.

PERITONITIS.—Puerperal Fever, Low Fever of Childbed, Uterine Phlebitis, Metritis, Metro-Peritonitis. This disease consists of acute inflammation of the peritonæum with typhoid fever. It is characterized by violent pain in the abdomen, increased by the slightest pressure, with general feverishness, and usually occurs soon after parturition. The ordinary allopathic treatment in this disease is not only horrid, but horridly murderous—bleeding, calomel, large doses of opium, etc., with hot flannel and turpentine or heavy bags of hop poultices to the abdomen. No wonder three-fourths of these poor patients die, victims to

"The deadly virtues of the healing art."

It should be treated precisely as I have recommended for Onteritis. I have treated many cases hygienically, as have other physicians of our school, and none of us have ever had any difficulty in curing them in a few days, *where there had been no bleeding* or *drug treatment* before we took the patient in hand.

PERTUSSIS.—Bex Convulsiva, Kin-Cough, Chin-Cough, Kind-Cough, Hooping Cough, Whooping Cough. The cough consists of several expirations, followed by a sonorous inspiration, returning periodically, with longer or shorter intervals. The disease is contagious, and rarely affects the individual the second time. The treatment must be adapted to the "grade" or degree of the attending feverishness, as in cases of pneumonitis. In mild cases a daily ablution, with a plain and rather abstemious dietary are all the attention required; but when the lungs are greatly engorged, or the pulmonary mucous membrane much inflamed, evinced by soreness, heat, laborious breathing between the paroxysms of coughing, and difficult expectoration, the full warm bath should be given, and if the fever "rises," after it, the wet-sheet pack or tepid ablution should be resorted to. When the heat and pain are continuous in the chest, the chest-wrapper or wet towels should be applied. Warm water may be taken to relieve the cough and expectoration, when the mucus is viscid and tenacious. In all cases the bowels must be kept free, and the diet must be light and sparing. Nearly all of the complications and dangers of the disease are owing to engorged stomachs and constipated bowels.

Pestilence.—Any malignant and prevalent disease.

Pestis.—Plague. In the middle ages this malady prevailed so extensively and fatally as to receive the appellation of "The Black Death," "The Black Mortality," etc. See Plague.

Petechiæ.—Puncticula. Small spots resembling flea-bites, which appear upon the skin in the course of putrid fevers. They are signs of great putrescency and exhaustion.

Phagedæna.—Sloughing of the mouth, Hospital Gangrene, Boulimia, Watery Cancer, an eating or corroding Ulcer. This affection requires the coldest applications locally, with prompt measures for the purification of the whole mass of the blood. Free ventilation, and an airy, light apartment are indispensable.

Phalangosis.—Trichiasis.

Phantasia.—Delirium, Disordered Imagination.

Phantasm.—Phantom, False Appearance, Hallucination.

Pharyngitis.—Cynanche Pharyngea, Inflammation of the Pharynx.

Pharyngitis, Apostematosa.—Abscesses of the Pharynx.

Pharyngitis, Diptheritic.—Membranific or Diptheritic Inflammation of the Throat; Cynanche Maligna.

Pharyngocele.—Prolapsus of the Œsophagus. An enlargement of the upper part of the gullet, in which the food sometimes lodges. It is owing to a relaxed condition of the mucous membrane, caused by inflammation or chronic con-

10

gestion. Cold water gargles, bits of ice, and a dry, abstemious dietary, comprise the especial remedial resources.

PHARYNGOPHLEGIA.—Paralysis of the Pharynx or Œsophagus. It may be a part of a general paralytic condition. In acute disease it indicates approaching dissolution.

PHENOMENA.—In pathology, the term includes all the symptoms or signs of disease.

PHIMOSIS.—Stricture of the Prepuce. A preternatural narrowness of the opening of the prepuce, preventing it from being retracted behind the *corona glandis*. It may be congenital, or caused by inflammation or swelling, as in syphilis. When cold applications will not overcome, circumscision, or a division of the prepuce, must be resorted to.

PHLEBISMUS.—Turgescence of the Veins.

PHLEBITIS.—Inflammation of a Vein. It often follows blood-letting, the pain and swelling extending from the wounded part to the neighboring parts of the venous system, and characterized by a knotty, tense, painful cord along the course of the principal vein, with more or less feverishness Cold applications are required.

PHLEGM.—Pituita. Stringy mucus, expectorated or vomited.

PHLEGMASIA.—Inflammation.

PHLEGMATIA, DOLENS.—Dolens Puerperarum. See Milk Leg.

PHLEGMON.—Boil; Suppurating inflammation of the areolar texture. It requires only cold wet cloths.

PHLEGMONOUS INFLAMMATION.—*Active* or *entonic* inflammation, in contradistinction to *erysipelatous, erythematic, passive,* or *atonic* inflammation.

PHLOGISTIC.—Inflammatory. This te:m *should* be limited to entonic inflammation.

PHLOGOSIS.—Inflammation.

PHLYCTÆNA.—Phlyctis, Phlysis. Accumulation of serous fluid under the epidermis.

PHOTOPHOBIA.—Intolerance of Light, Nyctalopia.

PHOTOPSIA.—False perception of Objects. Pressure on the eye-ball, congestion of the brain, and inflammation of the retina, are often accompanied with the recognition of sparks, flashes of fire, luminous balls, etc. Similar appearances are often noticed in the incipient stage of amaurosis. See Retinitis.

PHRENITIS.—See Cephalitis.

PHRENZY.—Phrenitis.

PHTHEIRIASIS.—Lousy Disease; Lousiness.

PHTHISIS.—Decline, Tabes, Consumption, Phthisic, Gradual Emaciation.

PHTHISIS, PULMONALIS.—See Consumption.

PHYMA.—Phlegmon, Boil, Anthrax.

PHYMOSIS.—Phimosis.

PHYSCONIA.—Pot-belly, Swag-belly, Pendulous Abdomen.

PHYSEMA, PHYSESIS.—See Tympanites.

PHYSOCELE.—Hernia Ventosa. An emphysematous tumor of the scrotum, or intestinal hernia.

PHYSOMETRA.—Uterine Tympanitis; Inflation of the Womb Collection of air in the uterus. It is connected with some form of menstrual disorder, and the treatment must be regulated accordingly.

PIMELOSIS.—Fatty Degeneration; applied to certain morbid states of the liver and kidneys. The ordinary process of fattening animals, or human beings, tends directly to produce this condition of those organs.

PIT, PITTING.—Pock Mark.

PITYRIASIS.—Dandriff, Dandruff, Tinea Furfuracea. An unimportant affection, consisting in the formation of irregular patches of thin scales on the surface, which repeatedly exfoliate. It indicates a slight defect in the functions of the cutaneous emunctory, or a too viscid condition of the blood, and is remediable by a daily ablution and a proper diet.

PLAGUE.—Pestis, Black Death. ° This is a malignant typhus of the putrid form. It is attended with glandular swellings, ulcerations and carbuncles, and hence the term, *Carbuncular Exanthem.* The Plague is nothing more nor less than the extreme manifestation of putrid typhus fever. All of the leading symptoms—black tongue, fetid breath, offensive excretions, burning pain in the epigastrium, and foul eruptions, etc.,—indicate extreme grossness of the body and putrescency of the blood. It has thus far been the most fatal fever which has ever prevailed extensively, the deaths having been more than two-thirds of all the cases. In the fourteenth, fifteenth, and sixteenth centuries, more than one hundred millions of the human race died of it. For the treatment, see Fever, Putrid.

PLAGUE, COLD.—The term has been applied to low states of the system in pneumonia, and in various fevers, where the hot stage—" the stage of reaction "—was absent or slight.

PLETHORA.—Repletion, Fullness. Medical authors give us two varieties of plethora, sanguine and nervous ; the former being the condition of superabundance of blood, and indicated by turgescence and redness of the surface, and the latter being the condition of superabundance of serous fluid, indicated by fullness with paleness of the surface. In both cases there is excessive alimentation, or defective depuration, or both. When the retained excrementitious matters are so accumulated as to render the blood very thick, gross and putrescent, the individual is liable on the application of the most trivial exciting causes, to fatal congestions of the brain or lungs. Such persons often die very suddenly of an "apoplectic stroke ;" usually termed, however, "visitations of God." Plain, dry, solid food in spare quantity, with abundant exercise, and a daily bath, are infallible remedies.

PIEUMONIA.—Pneumonia.

PLEURALGIA.—Pleurodyne, Pleurodynia, Stitch in the Side, Pain in the Side, False Pleurisy. This disease is often mistaken for pleurisy. It is a rheumatic or spasmodic affection of the intercostal or other muscles of the chest; the pain is increased on inspiration, and augmented by pressure, and there is more or less cough; dyspnœa sometimes exists. It may be distinguished from pleurisy, or pneumonitis, by the absence of fever. Warm fomentations, followed by the wet-girdle, will invariably remove it.

PLEURISY.—Pleuritis.

PLEURITIS.—Inflammation of the Pleura. This cannot be, and need not be, distinguished from *Pneumonitis*, of which it is really a part.

PLEURITIS, BRONCHIALIS.—Bronchitis.

PLEURODYNE, PLEURODYNIA.—Pleuralgia, which see.

PLEUROPNEUMONIA, PLEUROPERIPNEUMONY.—Inflammation of the Pleura and Lungs. These terms have been applied to co-existent pleurisy and pneumonia; and has lately been employed to designate a disease which has been very fatal among cattle in some parts of New England, and still more extensively fatal among hogs in the Western States. The real disease is, however, in all the cases to which these terms have thus far been applied, nothing more nor less than typhoid pneumonia, of very low diathesis.

PLEUROTHOTONOS.—Tetanus, with incurvation backward. See Tetanus.

PLICA.—Matted Hair; interlacing, twisting and agglutination of the hair. This affection has been endemic in Poland, Lithuania, and other parts of Northern Europe. Inattention to cleanliness is no doubt the essential cause; and this fact sufficiently indicates the remedial plan.

PNEUMATHORAX.—See Pneumothorax.

PNEUMAPOSTEMA.—Abscess in the Lungs; Apostematous Phthisis. See Consumption.

PNEUMONIA.—Pneumonitis.

PNEUMONITIS.—Pneumonia; Inflammation of the Lungs. This is one of the least dangerous of all the diseases which are really serious; yet, under the ordinary drug treatment, the mortality is enormous. More than fifty deaths per week have occurred in New York, not one in ten of whom would, in my opinion, have died had there been no physician in attendance. This may be said to be a *mere* opinion; but it is corroborated by the facts that deaths of pneumonitis are rare when the patients take no medicine at all, and that the physicians of the Hygienic school, who have treated hundreds of cases in this city, have not yet lost the first patient.

Pneumonitis is manifested in three forms: 1. *Phlegmonous Inflammation* of the lungs, with *Synochal or Inflammatory Fever;* this is commonly termed, simply, *Pneumonia.* 2. *Erysipelatous Inflammation*, with *Putrid Typhoid Fever;* this form is usually called *Bilious Pneumonia.* 3. *Erysipelatous Inflammation*, with *Nervous Typhoid Fever.* This form has been denominated, *Peripneumony notha.* The term Pleuropneumonia has been commonly applied to severe cases of the second or putrid variety, while the term *Congestive* is not unfrequently applied to severe cases of the third variety. The phrase, *Malignant Typhoid Pneumonia*, has been applied to severe cases of both the second and third variety. The "Typhoid Pneumonia," of which so many of our soldiers are reported to have died during our gigantic war, was of the second variety.

Pneumonitis may be known by a fixed pain in the chest, with sense of weight and heat in the lungs, cough, difficult breathing, expectoration, and fever.

Entonic Pneumonitis is characterized by strong pulse, white tongue, florid surface, whitish expectoration, and uniform heat and dryness.

Putrid Typhoid Pneumonitis may be known by the darker coat of the tongue, fetid breath, offensive excretions, crimson surface, dark or bloody expectoration, and, in malignant cases, dark spots or blotches on the skin.

In *Nervous Typhoid Pneumonia* the sputa is copious and frothy; the coat of the tongue is light colored without red edges; the redness of the face is more like the flush of hectic than the florid color of the *entonic*, or the crimson color of the *putrid* form; while the superficial heat is unequal, and the surface disposed to partial sweats.

So far as the constitutional disturbance, or fever, is concerned, the treatment should be precisely the same as for the corresponding forms of simple fever. In the *entonic* variety the wet-sheet pack is incomparably superior to all other bathing processes. It should be employed daily, with tepid ablutions two or three times a day in addition. The chest should bo kept constantly covered with cold wet cloths; the bowels should be kept free with enemas of tepid water; the patient may be allowed cold water or ice *ad libitum;* and abstinence from all food must be the rule without any exception, until the breathing becomes free, the expectoration easy, and the violence of the fever materially abated.

In treating the *putrid* variety all the rules must be observed which I have mentioned under the head of putrid-fever. (See Fever, Putrid.) In many cases the wet-sheet pack will be advisable, after the hot stage is fully developed; and in all cases the whole surface should be sponged with moderately cool water whenever the heat of the surface rises much above the normal standard. Cold drinks and ice may be allowed freely; and towels wet with tepid, cool, or cold water should be applied to the chest as long as there is preternatural external heat. As there is always a tendency to congestion of the brain and delirium, the head must bo kept cool, and the room well ventilated. The bowels must be moved freely at the outset with enemas of tepid water, and afterwards whenever there is fullness, weight or uneasiness in the abdomen from fecal matters.

In the *nervous* variety, the condition of the system is that of debility rather than grossness, and the whole plan of treatment must be mild, and directed more especially to balancing the circulation. The pack is seldom advisable, and very cold baths are never proper. When the cold stage is prolonged, or the extremities cold, hot bottles should be placed to the feet and sides. After the fever is fairly developed on the surface, tepid ablutions should be employed two or three times during each twenty-four hours; and if the breathing is laborious, or expectoration difficult, fomentations should be applied to the chest.

PNEUMORRHAGIA.—Hæmoptysis.

PNEUMOTHORAX.—Accumulation of air in the cavity of the pleura. It is generally, if not always, accompanied with tuberculation or inflammation.

POCK.—A Pustule of Small-pox.

POCK, KINE.—Vaccina.

POCKMARK.—Pock-hole, Pock-fretten. The *pit* or *pitting* which remains after a small-pox pustule.

POISONING.—The condition occasioned by venoms, viruses, malaria, drugs, banes, and all foreign substances. The plan of curing diseases by the administration of poisons, *alias* medicines, is simply a poisoning process from first to last— *Poisonopathy*, and nothing else. Drugs are said to act on the system *physiologically* when taken from the apothecary shop and prescribed by the physician, and to act *pathologically* when taken from any source, or swallowed accidentally, or when administered in "excessive doses" by medical men. This is a distinction with a very curious difference. And when the people can understand the simple truism that poison *is* poison, and that the effects of all poisons are *toxicological* purely, no matter what are the technicalities employed, there will be an end of "the greatest curse of the civilized world"—drug medication.

POLYDIPSIA.—Excessive Thirst. It is symptomatic in most febrile and inflammatory diseases. Nine-tenths of all the water ordinarily drunk by human beings is to assuage morbid thirst, induced by improper food and irritating condiments. Those who live physiologically have occasion to drink very little water.

POLYOPSIA.—Multiple Vision.

POLYPHAGIA.—Voracity.

POLYPHISIA.—Flatulence.

POLYPUS.—A tumor of a mucus, fleshy or scirrhous character which forms on the mucous membrane, and has some resemblance to certain zoophites. Polypi are more frequently found in the nasal fossæ, pharynx, and uterus.   They may be soft, spongy, or vesicular.   They may be removed by ligation, cauterization, excision, or extirpation, according to their nature and situation.

POLYSARCIA.—Corpulency, Obesity.   DUNGLISON recommends "a severe regimen."   It cannot be too mild; but it should be strictly physiological.   Children are often said to be excessively fat "in spite of every care."   It is because they do not have the *right* care.   Children who are properly fed never become so.

POLYURESIS, POLYURIA.—Diabetes.

POMPHOLYX.—Bullæ or Blebs.   See Pemphygus.

PORRIGO.—Scurf or Scall in the Head.   There are many varieties of this affection, but each is characterized by a pustular eruption of some kind, unaccompanied with fever. They are among the numerous manifestations of the scrofulous diathesis, or some other cachexy, and are more frequently the effects of the *medicines* which their parents have taken, particularly mercury, iron, and antimony, than is commonly supposed.   Cleanliness of the part, and general purification of the system, comprise the essential medication.

PORRIGO, DECALVANS.—Limited or Partial Baldness.   Cut the hair short, wet the whole scalp with cold water, morning and evening, using also gentle friction, or "shampooing." Hot viands, salt and pepper, are especially injurious to such patients.

PORRIGO, FAVOSA.—Scabies of the Head, Honey-Comb Scall, Tetter.   The eruptions are pea-sized, and appear on the body, and extremities also.

PORRIGO, FURFURANS.—An eruption of small achores, the fluid of which concretes and separates in scale-like exfoliations.

PORRIGO, LARVALIS.—Crusta Lactea; Milky Scall.   An eruption of numerous minute white achores on a red surface, which break and discharge a viscid fluid, which becomes incrusted in a thin, yellowish, or greenish scab.   The eruption

10*

appears at first on the forehead and cheeks, and is almost wholly confined to infants. The mother, if nursing the child, should look well to her own dietetic and other habits.

PORRIGO, LUPINOSO.—This variety consists of patches of minute pustules which terminate in dry scabs, resembling lupine seeds.

PORRIGO, SCUTULATA. — Granulated Tinea, Scalled Head, Ringworm of the Scalp. In this form the eruption commences with clusters of small, yellow pustules, which soon scab off. It is one of the most unmanageable varieties of porrigo. DUNGLISON says, "The whole tribe of stimulating ointments may be used in succession." I would advise that the "whole tribe" be thrown into the sea. The practice of *curing* cutaneous eruptions with lead, zinc, tar, mercurial, antimonial, sulphur, etc., etc., ointments and lotions, is wrong in theory and disastrous in effect. The disease may disappear on the surface, but it will exist in a more insidious and more injurious form in the internal organs. I have always succeeded in curing this affection by proper bathing and strict attention to the general regimen.

PREGNANCY, FALSE.—Moles, hydatids, polypus tumors, etc., which have formed in the cavity of the uterus, have received this appellation.

PRESBYTIA.—Long-Sightedness. A condition of vision in which near objects are seen confusedly, while those at a distance are clearly distinguished. Convex glasses will remedy the defect.

PRIAPISMUS.—Painful and prolonged erection without sexual desire. It is symptomatic of constipation, local inflammation, inordinate accumulation of urine, the irritation occasioned by acrid drugs, cantharides, etc. Tepid, but not very cold water, will in due time relieve it. The bowels should be freely evacuated, and all sources of irritation or constipation carefully avoided.

PROCIDENTIA.—Prolapsus.

PROCTOCACE.—Gangrenous inflammation of the rectum,

which is said to be common in Peru, and the neighborhood of Quito and Lima, on the Honduras and Mosquito coasts, in Brazil, and on the Gold coast. It has been attributed to bad food and spices.

PROCTOCELE.—Prolapsus Ani; Falling of the Fundament. Inversion and prolapsion of the mucous coat of the lower bowel. It is owing to relaxation, and may be restored by cool or cold hip-baths, enemas of a small quantity of cold water, or the introduction of small pieces of ice into the rectum, with due attention to the general health.

PROCTORRHŒA.—Hæmorrhois.

PROFLUVIUM.—Flux. A term applied to morbid discharges.

PROLAPSUS.—Procidentia, Prolapsion, Delapsus, Protosis; a falling down.

PROLAPSUS ANI.—See Proctocele.

PROLAPSUS UTERI.—Falling of the Womb; A displacement of the organ downward, or a descent from its normal position. This is a very prevalent abnormal condition. Its remote causes are constipation, sedentary habits, emmenagogues or "forcing" medicines, drastic purgatives, etc. The most prominent symptom is a sense of weight or bearing down, which is increased on standing or walking. A digital or speculum examination will readily determine the degree of the prolapse. The restorative plan must comprehend not only the reposition of the organ, but the invigoration of the whole muscular system, and especially the contractile tissue of the utero-vaginal region, so that it may be afterwards retained in the normal position. The multitudinous surgical processes and mechanical appliances which are usually resorted to, have done immense mischief; and it would be an incalculable blessing to womankind, and indirectly to mankind, also, if the whole catalogue of inventions and contrivances, called "pessaries," and "abdominal supporters," could be discarded at once and forever.

When the prolapsis is slight, no other local treatment is necessary than hip-baths, vaginal injections, and abdominal manipulations to remove the causes of inflammation, and restore tone to the relaxed muscles and membranes. In severer cases, when the organ is very low down in the passage, and when the os uteri protrudes externally, mechanical treatment is generally indispensable. The prolapsed organ should be pushed gently yet firmly upward—the patient meanwhile in the recumbent or horizontal position—and if the relaxation is extreme, a piece of fine, compressed sponge may be introduced (most conveniently through a cylinder or speculum,) and allowed to remain for a few hours. The patient should continue to rest for an hour or two after each reposition (which may be repeated daily or weekly according to the degree of relaxation,) and while in this position, the abdominal muscles should be manipulated by the attendant—rubbing, kneading, percussion, etc. In most cases, and especially when there is spinal curvature, or great weakness in the back, or inability to sit long in the erect position, an additional benefit will be derived from turning the face and spatting, rubbing, and kneading the muscles of the back. Hip-baths of a mild temperature—75° to 90°—vaginal injections and the wet-girdle, should be employed with a freedom proportioned to the local heat and irritation. In a majority of cases, there will be more or less inflammation of the mucous membrane—vaginitis—and when this is attended with much heat and pain, very cold injections, or pieces of ice introduced immediately after each reposition, will be serviceable.

Ulcerations of the os uteri are often found in connection with prolapsus. When they are superficial they readily heal when the inflammation subsides, or soon after the congestion is removed. When they are deep, with irregular, indurated, or corroding edges, they should be cauterized with nitrate of silver, or sulphate of zinc. The caustic should come in contact only with the part which is to be destroyed. The object is to destroy the abnormal edge or surface, so that healthy granulations may start from the sound tissue. When the ulcers are very deep, or their edges very thick, the caustic may have to be repeated several times. No harm will arise from the application of caustic agents to any required extent, if the treatment is properly attended to in other respects. The practice, as the manner of some is, of injecting strong caustic solutions over the whole vaginal mucous membrane, cannot be too strongly reprobated. I have known the health, happiness, and usefulness of several ladies ruined in this way.

No cases require a more strict and persevering regimen, so far as the dietary is concerned. Mushes must be eaten sparingly; milk, butter, cheese, puddings, and flesh-meat must be wholly abstained from. I have known poor women bedridden for years, with a prospect of continuing so for many years longer, and, probably, for the rest of their lives, because their own morbid sensations, and their own family physicians, told them that, *they could not live without meat.*

PROLAPSUS, UVULÆ.—See Staphylœdema.

PROLAPSUS, VAGINÆ.—Protrusion of the upper part of the vagina into the lower. The treatment is substantially the same as for prolapsus uteri. For a fuller explanation of these subjects, illustrated with plates, see the author's work, "Uterine Diseases and Displacements."

PROSPHYSIS.—Adhesion of the Eyelids.

PROSTRATITIS.—Inflammation of the Prostrate Gland.

PRURIGO.—An eruption of the papulæ of nearly the same color as the adjoining cuticle, accompanied with severe itching.

PRURITIS.—Gargle, Itching, Prurigo.

PSORA.—Scabiola, Itch, Scratch, Physis. The eruption of very minute pimples, pustular, vesicular, papular, intermixed, and alternating, itching intolerably, and terminating in scabs. It is probably caused by an insect of the genus *acarus*. Sulphur, hellebore, potash, muriate of ammonia, will destroy the insect; but water and coarse towels have always proved efficient in my practice.

PSORIASIS.—Scaly Tetter, Dry Scall, Scabies Sicca. This disease occurs in many forms, some of which are called *Baker's Itch, Grocer's Itch, Washer-woman's Scall, Psora agria.* This disease is a cutaneous affection, consisting of patches of rough, amorphous scales, continuous or of indefinite outline. The skin is generally extremely irritable and tender, and the bathing should in most cases be of water of a very mild temperature.

PTERYGION, PTERYGIUM.—Onyx, Pyosis, Unguis, Onglet. A varicose excrescence of the conjunctiva, whence it extends over the cornea. It will usually disappear soon after the inflammation subsides; if not, it can be removed with the scissors.

PTOSIS IRIDIS.—Hernia of the Iris, Iridoptosis, Prolapsus of the Iris. A protrusion of the iris through a wound of the cornea.

PTYALISM, PTYALISMUS.—Salivation.

PUERPERAL CONVULSIONS.—Convulsions occurring during or near parturition. Constipation or plethora are the most frequent causes. See Convulsions, Puerperal.

PUERPERAL FEVER.—Childbed Fever. See Peritonitis.

PUFFINESS.—Inflation, Sufflation. A soft intumescence without redness, occasioned by accumulation of serum, air, or extravasated blood, into the areolar texture. In different cases cold, tepid, warm, or hot water, may be the best application.

PUKING.—Vomiting, Regurgitation. See Emesis.

PULMONIA.—Pneumonia, Phthisis Pulmonalis.

PUNCTICULA.—Petechiæ.

PUOGENIA.—Pyogenia.

PURBLINDNESS.—Myopia.

PURGATION.—Catharsis. The term is applied to diarrhœa or cholera, when induced by what are called cathartic or purgative *medicines*. Probably there is no class of drug medicines which do so much mischief as this. Nearly all persons are taking them more or less, while every drug doctor prescribes them more or less in almost every case of disease he treats. Next to eating their way into premature graves, the great error of mankind is in purging themselves to death.

PURPURA.—Porphyra. Livid spots on the skin from extravasated blood, as in putrid fevers, scurvy, etc.

PURPURA, SIMPLEX.—Petechial Scurvy.

PURPURA, HÆMORRHAGICA.—Scorbutus, Land Scurvy, Purples. A putrescent state of the blood, characterized by livid or purplish spots, often in stripes or patches, irregularly scattered over the body and extremities, with occasional hemorrhages from the mouth, nostrils, or viscera, and great debility and depression of spirits. Abundance of pure air, simple food, with a large proportion of fruits, of vegetables, and strict abstinence from greasy food and salted meats, are the remedies.

PURPURA, NAUTICA.—Sea Scurvy. In this form of scurvy there are spots of different hues; the teeth are loose; the gums spongy and bleeding; the breath is fetid; the debility is universal and extreme. The treatment is the same as in the preceding case.

PURSINESS.—Short-windedness; Dyspnœa with Obesity.

PURULENCE, PURULENCY.—Pus, Suppuration

PUSTULATION.—The Formation of Pustules. The process is often resorted to as a remedial measure, on the principle of *counter irritation*, for which tarter emetic is commonly employed.

PUTREFACTION.—Rottenness, Putrid Fermentation. Decomposition of dead organic substances. *Antiseptics*, as salt, nitre, alcohol, charcoal, etc., have been used in medicine, on the theory that they would prevent the putrescent tendency of the fluids and solids of the body. But the theory is erroneous, and the practice pernicious.

PUTRID.—Gross, Putrescent; tending to Putrefaction. The term is applied to certain states of the system in low fevers and passive inflammations, in which the excretions are very offensive, and exhale an odor of putridity, as in typhus, plague, confluent small-pox, malignant scarlatina, black measles, etc.

PUTRID FEVER.—See Fever, Putrid.

PYÆMIA.—Pyohæmia.. An alteration and depravation of the blood by an intermixture of pus.

PYORRHŒA.—A Discharge of Pus.

PYREXIA.—Fever.

PYROSIS. — Cardialgia Sputatoria, Water-qualm, Black-water, Waterbrash. A hot sensation in the stomach, with eructations of an acrid, burning liquid. It is a common symptom of indigestion. It may be relieved by warm water-drinking, and can be cured by restoring the healthy condition of the digestive organs.

PYURIA.—Discharge of Purulent Urine. It occurs in cases of renal calculi, and in organic diseases of the bladder.

QUARTAN.—An intermittent fever whose paroxysms recur every fourth day.

QUEASINESS.—Nausea.

QUINIALIS.—Though this term is not found in the medical lexicons, I introduce it here for a purpose. I mean by it the state or condition of torpor and exhaustion in the whole nervous system which is induced by large or long continued doses of quinine. Dimness of vision, dullness of hearing, a sense of langor and lassitude, with torpidity of the liver, and a depression of the spirits, are the most obvious symptoms. A buzzing in the head, or ringing in the ears, or sense of constriction in the epigastrium, are regarded by physicians as evidences that the drug has "taken full effect"—an effect, however, whose consequences are as mischievous as they are lasting. Nothing can be more absurd than the notion almost universally entertained that quinine has some specific virtue or property of "neutralizing" or "counteracting" malaria. It may indeed prevent or cure (in the drugopathic sense) ague and fever, but it does it by preventing the system from expelling it, and therefore leaves the poison within. A sufficient number of such cures are sure death to the patient. A late author, in the Philadelphia *Medical and Surgical Reporter* has capped the climax of absurdity, by expatiating on the virtues of quinine in "*preventing*" malaria!

QUININISM.—Quinism, Cinchonism, Quininismus. All of these terms are found in DUNGLISON's Medical Dictionary, and are thus defined : " The aggregate of encephalic or neuropathic phenomena induced by over doses of quinine."

QUINSY.—Cynancho Tonsillaris, Tonsillitis, Inflammation of the Tonsils. It is easily recognized by the heat, redness, pain and swelling of glands. It is accompanied with continued fever, commonly of the entonic diathesis ; but sometimes the local inflammation is of the erysipelatous character and the corresponding fever of the atonic diathesis. In the latter case the disease is termed, *Typhoid or Malignant Quinsy.* Cold wet cloths around the throat, iced-water or ice in the mouth, with tepid ablutions when the fever is typhoid, and the wet-sheet pack when the fever is entonic, are the remedial measures. If these measures are promptly applied in the early stage, the disease will terminate by resolution, but if it proceeds to suppuration, indicated by great swelling, with throbbing, pain and extreme difficulty of breathing and swallowing, and a softening of the tonsils, they should be opened and the matter evacuated.

QUOTIDIAN.—Occurring Daily.

QUOTIDIAN FEVER.—Every Day Intermittent.

RABIES CANINA.—Hydrophobia.

RACHIALGIA.—Lead Colic; Metallic Colic. See Colic, Metallic.

RACHIPHYMA.—Tumor Dorsi. A tumor on the back, or spine.

RACHISAGRA.—A gouty or rheumatic affection of the spine.

RACHITIS.—English Disease; Rickets. An affection characterized by swelling of the extremities, crookedness of the spine, prominent abdomen; crookedness of the long bones, large head, and often precocity of intellect. Damp, dark, ill-ventilated situations, with gross food and poisonous drugs,

---

are the predisposing causes. Rickets is one manifestation of the scrofulous diathesis, and is often inherited from feeble, consumptive, mercurialized, liquor-drinking, tobacco-using, and pork-eating parents. Tepid bathing, a pure atmosphere, plain food, exercise, active or passive, in the fresh air, and frequent exposure to sunshine, constitute the remedial plan; but in many cases little can be done except to palliate the patient's sufferings.

RACHOSIS.—Relaxation of the Scrotum. Frequent cold ablutions and friction are the specialities of treatment.

RADZYGE.—Norwegian Leprosy; a malignant Ulcer. It is probably a variety of Elephantiasis.

RALE.—Rattle, Rhonchus. Noise produced by air passing through mucus, of which the lungs are unable to free themselves. It is seldom observed except at the approach of death, and is then called "*the rattles*."

RAMOLLISSEMENT.—Softening of the Structures.

RANULA.—Frog-Tongue. A small tumor which forms under the tongue, in consequence of accumulation in WHARTON's duct. When cold applications will not remedy it, a portion of the cyst may be removed with the scissors.

RAPHAMIA.—A convulsive disease common in Germany and Sweden, and which has been attributed to the seeds of a species of *Raphanus*, being mixed with the corn. The convulsive actions are mostly in the limbs, and are attended with acute pain. On the whole, the disease very much resembles the milk-sickness of some of our Western States.

RASH.—Exanthem; Cutaneous Disease.

REACTION.—This term is misdefined in the medical dictionaries, and misapplied by the medical profession. DUNGLISON says, "It is a state of activity which succeeds the action on the nervous system of certain morbific influences." As "morbific influences" do *not* "act on the nervous system," the explanation is a failure. A correct definition would be, the direct action of the vital powers in the process of expelling a morbific agent through the surface. Stimulants, especially the alcoholic, are given in the cold stage of low fevers to "produce," or "bring about," *reaction;* and in many diseases of very low diathesis, as diptheria, spotted fever, congestive chills, etc., they are given through their whole course to "maintain" action or reaction. These facts show that stimulation, and what medical books term "reaction," are precisely the "state of activity," and that both are morbid processes or remedial efforts to expel poisons. The common notion of "reaction" is founded on a false doctrine of the modus operandi of medicine, and the common practice of administering stimulants is predicated on a false theory of the nature of disease; while both of these errors are traceable to a fundamental error, a false dogma of the relations of living and dead matter.

Rectitis.—Inflammation of the Rectum.

Red Tongue Fever.—See Fever, Red Tongue.

Regurgitation.—In pathology this term is applied to the *puking* or *possetting* of infants; and to the *rising* of fluids or solids into the mouth in the adult. It is generally caused by over-eating. Dyspetics are sometimes troubled with it. Some persons have the power of regurgitating the food or other contents of the stomach at any time, or "vomiting at pleasure."

Relapse.—The reappearance of a disease after convalescence.

Relapsing Fever.—See Fever, Relapsing.

Relaxation.—Flabbiness, or looseness of a structure or part. It is the opposite of tone, tonicity, contractility, etc.

Remission.—Applied to fever, it means a prominent yet partial subsidence of the hot stage of the paroxysm. In a more extended sense, it means the diminution of any symptom of disease.

Remittens Icterodes.—See Fever, Yellow.

Remittent Fever.—See Fever, Remittent.

Repletion.—Fullness, Plethora.

RESOLUTION.—Removal or disappearance of disease without structural lesion.

RETENTION.—Permanent accumulation of a solid or liquid substance in a canal or cavity intended for its excretion.

RETENTION OF THE MENSES.—The menstrual flux may be retained in the uterine cavity or vaginal canal in consequence of obstruction of the os uteri or imperforate hymen. The symptoms are, sense of weight or heaviness in the pelvis, increased at the monthly periods, with puffiness of the face, and swelling of the feet in the evening. A digital or instrumental examination may be necessary to determine the nature of the difficulty. When the os uteri is closed by concreted mucus, warm-water injections, and subsequently the introduction of the uterine probe or sound, will relieve it. If the hymeneal membrane is imperforate, it should be divided by a crucial incision.

RETENTION OF URINE.—The urine may accumulate in the bladder from strangury or spasmodic contraction of the sphincter muscles; from atony of the muscular fibers of the body of the organ; from the presence of tumors in the vicinity, or foreign bodies within the bladder obstructing the urethra; inflammation of the urethra or prostrate gland; stricture, etc. Retention is a frequent complication in low fevers, and in paralytic affections. The application of Spanish flies to the surface, in the form of blistering plaster, will often cause *spasmodic* retention, while opium and other narcotic medicines, when given in large doses, will cause *atonic* retention. The urine is sometimes allowed to accumulate in the bladder because of the inconvenience or indelicacy of voiding it, until the muscles are so distended as to lose their power of contraction. Alternate hot and cold applications will always relieve, except when the obstruction is mechanical. The warm sitz-bath—as warm as can be borne—for a few minutes, immediately followed by the cold; or hot fomentations to the abdomen, followed by a dash of cold water, or the application of cold wet cloths, will relieve in most cases. But if they fail, resort must be had at once to the catheter. When the bladder is found distended above the pubis, with violent pain, no time should be lost in the treatment, or rupture of the bladder might take place.

RETINITIS.—Inflammation of the Retina. The symptoms are, deep-seated pain in the eyeball; the appearance of flashes of light, balls of fire, and various luminous bodies; intolerance of light, and more or less feverishness. It demands prompt attention, or the function of the optic nerve may be destroyed, and vision lost forever. The patient's apartment should be darkened, but well ventilated; cold wet cloths kept constantly on the eyes and over the whole face; tepid hip-baths and hot and cold foot-baths should be taken once or twice a day, and the whole surface sponged with tepid water whenever there is preternatural heat. Careful attention should be paid to the bowels, which must be kept entirely free, and the dietary must be simple and very abstemious.

RETROCESSION.—Disappearance or metastasis of an inflammation, eruption, tumor, etc., from the outer parts of the body to the inner. The practice of curing external diseases by *repelling* them, *scattering* them away, or "*driving them in,*" by means of astringents and irritant ointments, lotions, etc., is very common with physicians, but very dangerous to their patients. Such "cures" invariably make a very bad matter very much worse.

RETROFLEXION OF THE UTERUS.—That condition of retroversion in which the organ is doubled upon itself, the os uteri and fundus being near each other at the lower part of the tumor. See Retroversion of the Uterus.

RETROVACCINATION.—Vaccination with matter obtained from the cow, after inoculating the animal with vaccine matter from the human subject.

RETROVERSION OF THE UTERUS.—Displacement of the organ backward, the fundus or body being toward the rectum, and the os, or mouth, toward the bladder. Enlargement or congestion of the organ itself, and relaxation of the surrounding parts, more particularly of the vaginal canal and the abdominal muscles, are the common predisposing causes. Violent exertions and a distended bladder are the usual exciting causes. There is a sense of weight and distress in the lower part of the pelvis, increased on standing or walking; often an inability to walk at all; with constipation or difficult defecation, in consequence of the pressure of the body of the uterus on the lower bowel. A digital examination detects a globular tumor low down in and on the posterior part of the passage, with the os, or mouth, anteriorly, and a greater or less concavity between them, as the retroversion is more or less complete. The treatment is in all respects the same as for *Prolapsus Uteri*, with the exception of the manipulations. After the inflammatory condition is removed and the muscular tone manifestly improved, the fundus is to be gently elevated with the finger, or some convenient instrument, as far as possible toward its normal position; and these efforts at reposition must be repeated once, twice, or thrice a week, until the organ will remain in the normal position. The patient must gradually accustom herself to more and more exercise of various kinds, particularly in walking.

REVULSION.—Antispasis. See Derivation.

RHACHIALGIA.—See Spinal Irritation.

RHACHITIS.—Rachitis.

RHAGADUS.—See Fissure.

RHENCHUS, RHENXIS.—Rattle, Snoring.

RHEUM.—Any thin, watery discharge from the mucous membranes or skin.

RHEUM, SALT.—Various forms of hepatic and eczematous eruptions are so called. It is also applied to a kind of chronic psoriasis; also to cutaneous affections of those who expose their hands to extremes of heat and cold, or immerse them in acid or metallic solutions. Cleanliness, a simple diet, and an equable temperature, are the essentials of treatment.

RHEUMA.—Catarrh, Diarrhœa, Rheumatism.

RHEUMA CATARRHALE.—Bronchitis, Influenza, Leucorrhœa.

RHEUMATISM. — Inflammation of the Joints. Rhematism differs from gout only in affecting primarily the larger joints; whereas, gout primarily affects the smaller joints. When several or both the large and small joints are affected, it is termed *Rheumatic Gout*, or *Gouty Rheumatism*, as the disease primarily affects the larger or smaller joints. Rheumatism may be *acute*, with regular fever; *subacute*, with irregular feverishness; or *chronic*, without febrile disturbance. The "seat," as it is improperly called, is in the muscles, or denser tissues of the joints. The principal forms of Rheumatism are the *Inflammatory*, *Articular*, *Spasmodic*, and *Chronic*. The first and second varieties, though both are acute and severe, are of opposite diathesis, but are strangely confounded in medical books, and hence, as a necessary consequence, sadly maltreated by most physicians.

Inflammatory Rheumatism is accompanied with *entonic fever*. The discriminating symptoms are white tongue, strong pulse, turgescence and florid redness of the whole surface; tenderness and heat of the whole surface; great pain, lameness, or soreness about the small of the back, increased on the slightest motion; in most cases the patient cannot stand, nor rise from the bed, nor be turned over, without excruciating pain. The joints are not greatly swollen. The treatment is precisely the same as for simple or entonic or inflammatory fever, with the addition of cold wet cloths to the joints whenever there is much swelling, heat, and pain. The wet-sheet pack, when the patient can be handled by experienced attendants or nurses, should be employed for an hour, toward the middle of the day, and again in the evening. When the heat of the surface is very great, double sheets should be used. When the patient cannot be moved without great distress, cool or cold ablutions should be employed with a frequency proportioned to the external heat. The bowels are always constipated, and should be freely moved with tepid enemas. In no febrile disease is abstemiousness in diet, or rather abstinence from food, more important. No food at all should be taken until the violence of the fever, and the swell-ing and pain of the joints has materially abated, and then nothing more than gruel in very moderate quantity, and a little good ripe fruit should be taken until convalescence is fairly established. By rigidly adhering to this plan, the dis-ease can always be brought to a favorable termination in a few days. I have rarely had a case in which the patient was not convalescent in one week; whereas, under the ordinary bleeding, irritating, blistering, opium, and mercurial treatment, patients generally linger for weeks, frequently for months, and are often, very often, made cripples for life—not by the disease, but by the treatment.

Articular Rheumatism is commonly termed *Rheumatic Fever*, or *Acute Rheumatism*, in medical writings. Some of the larger joints are more swollen than in the preceding form, but there is not the same tenderness of the skin, nor distress in the back; the patient can be much more easily moved; and, moreover, the fever is of the *atonic* diathesis, as indicated by frequent and not strong pulse, partial and irregular sweats, etc. In this form of rheumatism bleeding is even more dis-astrous, and, mistaking the *hard* for the *strong* pulse, and acuteness for entonic action, physicians generally bleed more freely in this form, than in the inflammatory, which practice seldom fails to shatter the constitution and render the patient a miserable invalid for life. But, worse even than this, are opiates, mercurials, blisters, hydriodate of potassa, colchicum, etc., etc., with which these unfortunates are dosed and drugged.

The wet sheet pack is the best *refrigerant* as long as the febrile heat is maintained on the surface. Tepid ablutions will accomplish the same object, though not so rapidly. When the heat of the surface is slight or irregular, a full warm bath should be administered. The swollen joints should be constantly "soaked" in cloths wet in the coldest water. In other respects the directions given in the preceding case will apply here. This form of rheumatism can always be cured within two weeks, by proper hygienic treatment. It is rarely "cured" drugopathically in less than six or eight weeks, to say nothing of the "cure" being ten-fold worse than the disease.

Spasmodic Rheumatism comprehends the various forms of the disease, attended with pain, stiffness, soreness, or cramping in the muscles, without heat, redness or swelling, as *sciatica*, lumbago, and certain anomalous or nondescript aches and pains, which have received the appellation of *Rheumatalgia*. What is called *muscular rheumatism* is more frequently the consequence of mineral drugs, especially mercury, than of any other cause; and the same may be said of a majority of the cases of *chronic* rheumatism extant.

In all of these cases the local treatment consists of hot fomentations, or the warm or vapor bath, to relieve pain and spasms, and due attention to the general health.

Chronic Rheumatism requires no speciality of treatment, except the application of wet bandages to the hot, swollen or inflamed joints. The *Hydro-Electrical, alias Electro-Chemical* baths, are excellent in most forms of chronic rheumatism, rheumatalgia, sciatica, etc.; not because they have any specific virtue or property to eliminate mercury or any other drug, as is pretended by certain charlatans, and believed by some chemists who ought to know better, but because they are efficient agents in promoting and maintaining circulation to the whole surface, and thereby accelerating the elimination of *all* impurities, effete matters, and foreign substances from the system.

RHINANCHONE.—Snuffles.

RHINITIS.—Inflammation of the Nose; Coryza.

RHINORRHAGIA.—Epistaxis.

RHONCHUS.—Rattle, Stertor, Snoring, Gurgling.

RHUMATALGIA.—Spasmodic Rheumatism.

RHUME.—Rheum.

RHYSIS.—Flux.

RICKETS.—Rachitis.

11

RIGIDITY.—Stiffness and Immobility of Fiber.

RIGOR.—Shivering, Chilliness.

RIGOR, MORTIS.—Death-Stiffening.

RINGWORM.—A variety of Herpetic Eruption. See Herpes.

RISING.—Regurgitation.

RISING OF THE LIGHTS.—Croup.

RONCHUS.—Snoring, Stertor.

ROSALIA.—Scarlatina.

ROSE DROP.—See Gutta Rosea.

ROSEOLA.—Rose Rash; Erysipelatous Efflorescence. It appears chiefly on the face, neck, and arms, in blushing patches, alternately fading and reviving, during dentition, in indigestion, chronic and subacute rheumatic affections, etc.

ROSEOLA, ACNOSA.—Gutta Rosea.

ROSEOLA, FICOSA.—Sycosis.

ROSEOLÆ.—Roseola; False Measles. An imaginary malady between scarlatina and measles.

ROT.—Eructation.

ROT, GRINDERS'.—See Asthma.

RUBEFACTION.—The process of reddening the skin, or the action occasioned by the application of acids, irritants, or stimulants to the skin. Mustard, vinegar, cayenne, alcohol, etc., are commonly employed. The effect is nothing more nor less than inflammation.

RUBEOLA.—Measles. The premonitory stage is marked by cough, sneezing, running at the nose, watery eyes, and other catarrhal symptoms. The rash, which appears from the third to the sixth day, is characterized by distinct, red, and nearly circular spots, increasing and coalescing, until they form small patches of an irregular figure, but somewhat resembling that of semicircles or crescents. The rash and fever usually decline after three or four days' continuance, and the disappearance of the eruption is followed by a desquamation of the cuticle.

Measles may be accompanied with the *entonic* or *inflammatory* fever, or with *putrid typhus*. In the former case the disease is *benign* or *common measles*, and in the latter case *malignant* or *black measles*. The treatment, as in all febrile diseases, must be regulated by the external temperature. If the determination to the surface is too great, the morbid matter will not be easily eliminated, because of the over-distention of the superficial capillaries; and if it be too feeble it will be retained in the system. All that is required in either case is to maintain the balance of circulation; and this means maintaining the heat of the skin as nearly as possible at the normal standard. When the eruption does not come out well and there is little heat at the surface, with oppression of the head, lungs, or distress in the region of the stomach, the warm bath should be given; but if the pulse is strong, the tongue white, the skin turgid and florid, and the heat and dryness uniform over the surface, tepid ablutions, or better still, the wet-sheet pack should be employed. When there is much cough, and pain in the lungs, with difficult breathing, in the *typhoid* form, fomentations to the chest, with hot bottles to the feet are proper; but if these occur in the *entonic* form, cold wet towels should be applied to the chest. In the majority of cases very little treatment, save quiet, fresh air, and due attention to cleanliness is required.

RUPIA.—Rhypia, Rhyparia, Atonic Ulcer. An eruption of large flattish blebs, which contain a fluid which becomes puriform and bloody, and which soon concretes into crusts, at the base of which are ulcers of variable depths. The part should be fomented, then well cleansed, the ulcers covered or filled with fine flour, retained by strips of adhesive plaster, and wet compresses applied over the whole.

RUPTURE.—Hernia.

SABURRA.—Sabura, Sordes, Foulness of the Stomach. The presence of vitiated bile, imperfectly digested aliment, and morbid excretions, are the causes; and fasting, with small draughts occasionally of pure water, is the remedy.

SACCULATED.—Encysted.

SAINT JOHN'S DANCE.—See Mania, Dancing.

SAINT VITUS' DANCE.—Chorea. See Mania, Dancing.

SALIVATION.—Sialismus, Sputum Oris, Sialorrhœa, Sialoze-mia, Ptyalism, Ptyalismus, Fluxus Salivæ, Flux de Bouche. Copious excretion from the salivary glands. It may be occa-sioned by acrid or irritating articles taken into the mouth, as tobacco, lobelia, yarrow, cayenne pepper, or by poisons re-ceived into the mass of the blood, as the mercurials.

When an increased flow of saliva is excited by the sight, smell, or thought of agreeable food, it is called *mouth-watering*. In this case the secretion has a mucilaginous and sweetish taste; but when the discharge from the salivary glands are provoked by the presence of poisons, or by anger, rage, fury, etc., the fluid is acrid and excoriating; it is then an *excretion*, and not saliva at all.

Mercurial salivation is one of the most horrible of the multi-tudinous, abominable effects of a false and murderous "healing art." The tongue is swollen, hot, painful, cracked, ulcerous, fills the throat almost to the extent of inducing suffocation, and often protrudes from the mouth, while a stream of acrid sanies, or sordes, issues from the mucous membrane; the gums are tender, fleecy and bleeding; the taste is nauseous and ap-perish; the breath foul; the nerves neuralgic; the muscles tremulous; the brain semi-delirious; while a low, wasting fever, with frequent and irregular pulse, tells of the destruc-tion going on within the domain of organic life, in the struggle of the vital powers to expel their deadly enemy—*the doctor's medicine!* No person after being once thoroughly salivated can ever have a sound constitution afterward; and many of the infirmities, deformities, taints, humors, scrofula, and other ca-chexias, owe their origin to the medicines which their father's took before they were begotten, or which were administered to their mothers before they were born.

Salivation is an inflammation of the mouth and salivary glands, of the *erysipelatous* or *passive* kind, with an accompanying fever of the *atonic* diathesis and *putrid* form—really *putrid typhus.* The local affection which mercury occasions in the mouth is precisely analogous to gonorrhœal inflammation of the genital organs, induced by the venereal virus; and in its effects on the system much the worse of the two. The treatment must be very mild and gentle. Very cold water must be avoided, and all violent disturbances, or shocks to body or mind, must be carefully guarded against. Patients under what is called "mercurial action" are liable, on a little exertion, as rising suddenly from the bed, walking across the room, etc., even after convalescence is considered as fairly established, to die almost instantly. The patient should be kept as quiet as possible, sponged with tepid or moderately warm water occasionally, the extremities kept warm, the head cool, sips of cool, but not very cold, water allowed frequently, and the mouth washed or gargled with the same. After the miserable patient has recovered sufficiently to be about, he may then begin to think of a radical cure, which is a course of treatment at some Hygienic establishment for a year or two, in order to get the mercurial medicine out of his blood, glands and bones.

SALTANS ROSA.—Urticaria.

SAND-BLIND.—Defective vision, in which small particles seem to float before the eyes. See Metamorphopsia.

SANGUINOLENT.—Tinged with Blood.

SANIES.—Ichor, Malignant Pus. A thin, serous fluid resembling an admixture of pus and blood, which is exhaled at the surface of foul ulcers.

SARCITIS.—Myositis.

SARCOCELE.—Schirrhus or Cancer of the Testicle. Extirpation of the organ is the only remedial resource, except in the very early stages, when the refrigerating treatment might be successful. See Cancer.

SARCOMA.—Sarcosis. Any excrescence having a fleshy consistence. Sarcomatous tumors are found in the mammary glands, testes, and other parts.

SARCOSTOSIS.—Osteo-Sarcoma.

SARDIASIS.—Canine Laugh; Risus Sardonicus.

SATURNISMUS.—Saturnine Cachexy; Lead-Poisoning.

SATYRIASIS.—Satyrismus. An irresistible desire in man for frequent sexual intercourse, with almost constant priapism. Irritant drugs, high seasonings, worms in the lower bowel, combined with constipated habits, and an inflammatory condition, are among the principal causes. Abstinence, or abstemious diet, and prolonged tepid hip-baths, a daily ablution, and active exercise or occupation, are the remedies.

SAUSAGE POISON.—Allantotoxicum. A poison developed in sausages made of blood and liver. Such food is extremely unwholesome, if not actually poisonous, under all circumstances.

SCABIES.—Psora.

SCABIES, FESORIA.—Itch of Animals. See Mange.

SCALE.—An opake and thickened lamina of cuticle.

SCALE, DRY.—Psoriasis.

SCALL.—Impetigo.

SCALLED HEAD.—See Porrigo Scutulata.

SCARIFICATION.—Small Incisions; the act of scarifying. An absurd and barbarous method of drawing blood, or of inducing counter-irritation, to which physicians frequently resort.

SCARLATINA.—Red Fever, Rash Fever, Scarlet Fever. This is the most common and prevalent of the eruptive fevers. No disease, unless it is consumption, can be named in which medical men have pursued more discordant and conflicting plans of practice; and all the statistics which can be gathered from the four quarters of the globe, will sustain the assertion which I make here, advisedly and deliberately; that the mortality has ever, and in all places, been precisely according to the potency of the drug medication. Well did Professor BARKER, of the New York Medical College, say to his class not long since: "The drugs which are administered for the cure of scarlet fever and measles, *kill* far more than those diseases do."

The characteristic symptoms of scarlatina are, a scarlet flush, about the second day of the fever, on the face, neck, and fauces, and spreading progressively over the body. It terminates in about one week. The tongue has a peculiar *strawberry* appearance, which has been regarded as pathognomonic.

The disease exists in three distinct forms: 1. *simple* or *mild scarlatina*, in which the fever is entonic or inflammatory, and in which the throat is unaffected. This form scarcely requires medication. An enema to free the bowels, and tepid ablutions whenever the external heat calls for it, are sufficient. 2. *Anginosa scarlatina*, in which the glands of the neck are much swollen, with typhoid fever of the nervous form. This form of the disease is much more serious, though scarcely dangerous, independent of treatment. The fever is more prolonged, generally continuing from nine to fourteen days, and requires more frequent and more thorough bathing. After the bowels have been moved freely, cold wet cloths should be applied around the neck; renewed as often as they become warm, and continued until heat and swelling abate. The wet-sheet pack is applicable to the hot stage of the fever daily, although frequent ablutions of tepid and cool water will be efficient. 3. *Malignant scarlatina*—sometimes called "putrid sore throat," and often confounded with the severer forms of *diptheria*—in which the fever is the putrid form of typhus, and the throat more or less ulcerated. In all severe cases of scarlatina, a single bleeding, an emetic, an antimonial sudorific, or a castor oil cathartic, if performed or administered when the vital powers are exerting all of their energies to carry the morbid matter to the surface, (and just as the eruption is about to take place,) is often as sure death as would be a dagger through the heart. Yet thousands are *finished* in this way annually, and the physicians call it "medical science," and the people think—nothing.

The general treatment for all forms of scarlatina is the same, due regard being had to the degree and kind of fever, as indicated by the external temperature. In some cases of the malignant variety, though there may be a sense of *stinging heat* of the surface complained of, the temperature will be thermometrically low, and the warm bath should be employed, to be followed, when the external heat rises, by tepid ablutions or the wet-sheet pack. Cold applications must be made around the throat and sips of iced-water or bits of ice frequently taken into the mouth. In very bad cases, pounded ice should be applied externally to the throat.

SCARLET FEVER.—See Scarlatina.

SCIATICA.—A neuralgic affection, characterized by pain along the course of the great sciatic nerve, extending from the hip or pelvic region to the leg and foot. Fomentations, followed by gentle friction, will relieve the pain. The malady is always symptomatic, and must be cured by restoring the general health.

SCIEROPIA.—Defect of vision in which objects appear darker than natural.

SCIRRHUS.—Scirrhosis, Carcinoma Simplex, Hard Cancer. Fibrous Cancer. A hard tumor, usually the first stage of true cancer. It is accompanied, in most cases, with shooting pains, and is generally somewhat irregular on its surface. In the early stage it can generally be arrested by repeated freezings. See Cancer.

SCLEROTITIS.—Inflammation of the sclerotic coat of the eye.

SCORBUTUS.—Scurvy. See Purpura.

SCRATCH.—Psora.

SCROFULA.—The Evil, Cruels, the King's Evil. The manifestations of scrofula are innumerable, constituting a large number of distinct diseases in the nosologies, all of which are treated of in this work under their respective heads. The *scrofulous diathesis* is a state of the system characterized by laxity and flabbiness of the muscular tissue, glandular swellings or indolent tumors, most frequently in the neck, suppurating slowly, and healing with difficulty. This diathesis is often induced in constitutions originally sound, by the free use of mineral medicines of which mercury and antimony (all honor to Surgeon-General HAMMOND, for expelling them from the supply tables of the United States armies,) are the most potent, and thence transmitted to their offspring. The ordinary habits of living, especially in the agricultural districts of the civilized world, where pork, ham, sausages, lard, hot biscuit—made hotter with saleratus—old cheese, dried beef, salted fish, strong cheese, etc., constitute the principal part of the dietary, are conducive to scrofula in its multitudinous forms. The more familiar diseases which are evidences of, or essentially modified by, the scrofulous diathesis, are rickets, caries of the bones, white swellings, hip-disease, lumbar abscess, tubercular consumption, etc. In the treatment of all forms of scrofula, pure air and abundant sunshine are of the first importance ; next in order is a healthful dietary, which should exclude flesh meat, and even milk, after the teeth are developed. Exercise, frequent, various, but not exhaustive, is next in order ; and last, though perhaps not least, is the daily ablution, which, for feeble persons, should always be of moderate temperature, and taken in a comfortably warm room.

SCROTOCELE.—Scrotal Hernia, Oscheocele.

SCURF.—Small Exfoliations of the Cuticle.

SCURVY.—Scorbutus.

SCURVY OF THE ALPS.—Pellagra.

SCYBALA.—Indurated Feces. Hard fecal matters which are discharged in round lumps.

SEA-SICKNESS.—See Nausea, Marina.

SEDATION.—The state of quietness or torpor occasioned by certain drugs which are called *sedatives*. They are nervines or narcotics, as musk, valerian, opium, henbane, etc. They are said to "allay morbid irritability ;" but if physicians would explain the rationale of this process, their patients most certainly would refuse to be *allayed* by such means.

SEDIMENT.—A deposit of something suspended in a liquid. Much attention has been paid to the sediment which is precipitated from the urine, as affording a rule of diagnosis, and an indication for treatment. In calculous affections the sediment contains various mucus, earthy and saline concretions; and in that state of the system, called *bilious*, there is a brany or brick-dust like deposit. In the latter case, the urine is also high-colored. The practice of analyzing the urine with the view of prescribing to its chemical elements, is absurd. It is the *cause* of those impurities to which the physician should direct his remedial resources. The way to "cure" calculous and biliary matters in the urine, is not to neutralize them by chemicals, which is only introducing additional impurities, but to stop the supply of the materials of which they are formed, viz: bad water and impure food. If this is done, the existing impurities will in due time be eliminated, and there will be a cure indeed.

SEIRIASIS.—*Coup de Soleil.*

SELF-ABUSE.—Masturbation.

SELF-LIMITED.—A modern epithet, applied to diseases which run a definite course, independently of medication, and, as Dr. BIGELOW, of Boston, says, "deriving laws from their own nature," terminate—*when their course is run.* The theory of self-limitation is founded on a false doctrine of the nature of disease. Disease, being remedial action, is limited to the accomplishment of the object in view—purification and reparation, or the available resources of the vital powers under the circumstances. A full discussion of this subject will be found in the author's large work, "Principles of Hygienic Medication."

SEMIPLEGIA.—Hemiplegia.

SHINGLES.—Herpes.

SHIP FEVER.—See Typhus.

SHOCK.—Concussion; sudden deprivation of Sensibility

SHORT-SIGHTED.—See Myosis.

SHUDDERING.—Slight spasmodic movements of the muscles, with a sensation of coldness.

SIBBENS.—Framboesia Scotica. An infectious disease, supposed to be venereal, in the mountainous parts of Scotland.

Some regard the affection as a complication of venereal disease and the itch. In the Orkneys, the term *sibbens* means itch. The peculiarity of the disease is the appearance of fungi, which resemble raspberries. Cleanliness and caustic are the remedies.

SIDERATIO.—Planet-Struck. The ancients applied this epithet to paralysis, apoplexy, gangrene, etc., on the supposition that the stars had some influence in inducing these maladies.

SIMULATED DISEASES.—Feigned Diseases.

SINGULTUS.—Hiccup, Hiccough.

SIRIASIS.—*Coup de Soleil.*

SLAVERING.—Drivelling; involuntary flow of saliva.

SLEEPLESSNESS.—See Insomnia.

SLEEP-WALKING.—See Somnambulism.

SLOWS.—Milk-Sickness.

SMALL-POX.—See Variola.

SNEEZING.—Convulsive motion of the expiratory muscles, by which the air is driven rapidly and sonorously through the nasal fossæ.

SNORING.—Rhonchus, Stertor. Noise made in the back part of the mouth and nasal fossæ during inspiration. Relaxed palate, an overloaded stomach, enlarged tonsils, and compression of the brain, as in apoplexy, may occasion it.

SNUFFLES.—Difficulty of breathing through the nose, owing usually to accumulated mucus, or swelling of the mucous membrane. Infants are quite liable to it. Warming the feet and oiling the interior of the nostrils will relieve it.

SOLIDISM.—The doctrine that all diseases are essentially owing to alterations in the solids of the body, or have their seat primarily therein, as opposed to *Humoral Pathology.* It is the prevailing medical doctrine. When it is understood that impurities in the fluids are the principal *causes* of disease, and that the *action* of the solids in the process of expelling them constitute the *essence of disease,* these "pathologies" will have very little importance.

SOMNAMBULISM.—Lunatismus, Noctambulation, Sleep-Walking. Actions performed during sleep, and without the use of the external senses, similar to those which are performed during the wakeful period. The immediate causes are, congestion of the brain, indigestion, or any source of irritation which prevents quiet rest.

SOMNIUM.—Insomnium; a Dream. Confused and imperfect recognition of objects by the mind during disturbed or imperfect sleep. DUNGLISON, in his dictionary, says: "A confused assemblage, or accidental and involuntary combinations of ideas and images, which present themselves to the mind during sleep." This is a very *confused* definition, and, though agreeing with the prevailing metaphysics, does not quite square with sound philosophy. It is the mind which presents itself to the objects, and not the objects which present themselves to the mind. The "images" are *mental recognitions*, not extraneous entities. There is a world of delusion in this notion that external objects act on, make an impression on, or present themselves to the mind. Ideas do not present themselves to the mind; they are the exercises of the mind—mental recognitions, again.

SOMNOLENCY.—Sleepiness. It is sometimes an indication of congestion of the brain.

SORDES.—A dark, sanious matter discharged from ulcers; also foul matters in the stomach, or on the teeth, in low, putrid fevers.

SORE.—Ulcer.

SORE, BAY.—A cancerous disease, said to be endemic in the Bay of Honduras.

SORE MOUTH.—Stomatitis, Clergyman's Sore Throat, Throat-Ail. It is always symptomatic of diseased liver or indigestion. The practice of cauterizing the throat in these cases, with a solution of nitrate of silver, for months and years, with no regard to the primary malady or real cause, though very profitable to the physician, and very fashionable in the "upper circles," is the contrary of beneficial to the patient.

Stomatitis is often aggravated into *laryngitis*, and this to consumption, by this cauterizing process. If the digestive organs are properly medicated, the throat-ail will take care of itself.

SPANÆMIA.—Poverty of the blood. Some of the works on materia medica give us a class of medicines which *impoverish the blood!* They are called *Spanæmics*, a term which might with propriety apply to every article in the drug shop.

SPASM.—Involuntary and inordinate muscular contraction. The following tabular arrangement of spasmodic diseases, copied from the author's "Hydropathic Encyclopædia," may be convenient for reference:

Comatose Spasm.	Convulsion, Epilepsy, Hysterica.	Clonic Spasm.	Hiccough, Sneezing, Palpitation, Nictitation, Subsultus, Stretching.
Synclonic Spasm.	Tremor, Delirium Tremens, Shaking Palsy, St. Vitus' Dance Raphania, Barbiers.		
Suffocative Spasm.	Cough, Dyspnœa, Asthma, Laryngismus, Incubus, Sternalgia, Pleuralgia.	Constrictive Spasm.	Hydrophobia, Acrotismus, Tetanus, Locked Jaw, Cramp, Muscular Spinal Distortion, Muscular Stiff-Joint, Wry Neck.

SPERMATORRHŒA.—Nocturnal Emissions. This affection requires a rigidly simple dietary, and an entire abstinence from all irritating condiments; even milk and all its preparations, sugar and puddings, should be abstained from. When the temperature of the body is sufficient, a tepid ablution should be taken each morning, and, if there is not much emaciation, a hip-bath at about 80°, once or twice a day, is advisable. The wet-girdle, a part of each day, is applicable to those cases in which the liver is particularly inactive, or the bowels constipated, provided it can be worn without much chilliness. Exercise of either work or play is important. It should be frequent, varied, and, if possible, agreeable, but never very fatiguing. No cases require a stricter regimen or greater perseverance on the part of the patient. In some cases one, two, or three years are required for a cure, though many will recover in a few months, and some in a few weeks.

SPHACELUS.—Cold Mortification; total death of a part.

SPHRAGIDONYCHARGOCOMETA.—The beauty of technicality may be seen in this term, which has been applied to " a charlatan who adorned his fingers with rings to the very nails."

SPINAL IRRITATION.—Rachialgitis, Neuralgia Spinalis, Notalgia. DUNGLISON says: "A modern pathological view, which refers most nervous diseases to irritation of the spinal cord." Thousands of invalids are cupped, leeched, blistered, irritated, burnt, excoriated, and tortured, along the spine, or around the small of the back, in accordance with this " modern pathological view," but with most disastrous results so far as the patient is concerned. Affections of the lungs, liver, stomach, spleen, kidneys, uterus, etc., are often accompanied with tenderness of the spine, especially on pressure, near the origin of the nerves which are distributed to the diseased organs; and this tenderness is vaguely pronounced, " spinal irritation," and the poor patient is drugged, and bled, and cauterized, and perhaps also mercurialized, iodinized, antimonialized, ironized, etc., un'il utter prostration or unendurable neuralgia causes a respite in the medication. . Of hundreds of cases which have come under my professional notice of patients thus treated or maltreated for " spinal irritation," the real difficulty was obstruction, or chronic inflammation, or tuberculation, of some one or more of the internal organs, the spinal tenderness being a mere incident or s mptom. In relation to this symptom DUNGLISON says: " Such tenderness, however, by no means indicates the pathological condition in question, as it is often met with in those enjoying perfect health." I cannot imagine how " tenderness" of any kind, or in any place, can be consistent with *perfect* health, though I can easily understand how persons thus affected may not be *very* sick.

SPLENIC TUMOR.—Ague-Cake.

Splenitis.—Inflammation of the Spleen. Acute inflammation of the spleen is very rare. The symptoms are, pain, swelling and heat in the part, with general fever. The only special treatment required is the wet-girdle. Chronic inflammation of the organ is not uncommon, but the symptoms are very obscure. Obstruction and enlargement are still more frequent morbid conditions, and are accompanied with general nervous debility, great torpor of the bowels, weakness of the lower extremities, and depression of spirits. The required treatment is general, as for dyspepsia.

Splenization.—A condition of the lung in pneumonia, in which it resembles the spleen.

Splenocele.—Hernia formed by the Spleen.

Splenohæmia.—Congestion or hyperæmia of the Spleen. It occurs more or less in all entonic fevers, and especially the typhoid and intermittent forms.

Sporadic.—Diseases which occur independently of epidemic or contagious influence.

Spots, Red.—Rose Spots. They are common to all putrid fevers, and are most freqently seen on the chest and upper part of the abdomen.

Spotted Fever.—A form of *putrid typhus*, and should be treated as such. See Fever, Spotted.

Sprain.—A Wrench, Subluxation. Violent straining or twisting of the tissues surrounding the joints. The consequence is inflammation, and the result to be feared is permanent incurvation. The prompt and persevering application of cold water in any convenient manner, is sufficient in all ordinary cases. When there is great pain and tenderness, with little heat, hot fomentations, followed by cold compresses, are preferable. After the inflammation and tenderness have subsided, friction is useful to promote absorption and restore tone to the part.

Sputum.—Spit, Spittle. Excreted matter ejected from the mouth. Spitting is as much an abnormal process, a disease —*remedial effort*—as is coughing, sneezing, expectoration, or vomiting. Tobacco-users are *spitting their lives away*. Everything taken into the mouth, which occasions spitting, or which provokes the action of the salivary glands, except while food is being masticated or swallowed, cannot be otherwise than injurious.

SQUEASINESS.—Nausea.

SQUINTING.—Strabismus, Cross-Eyed, Squint-Eyed.

STAGNATION.—Accumulation and retardation of fluids.

STAMMERING.—Stuttering, Misenunciation. Imperfect articulation may be caused by constitutional defect, or acquired habits. In the latter, the training of a good elocutionist will generally effect a cure; and in the former, the defect may be greatly relieved, and not unfrequently cured. Speaking very slowly and deliberately, always taking care to keep the lungs well expanded, never undertaking to utter a sound when they are nearly collapsed, will be sufficient, in some cases, to effect a complete restoration. When the muscles of articulation are extremely irritable and spasmodic, speaking loudly and deliberately, with pebbles or other impediments in the mouth, has additional advantages. Mechanical instruments have been employed with advantage in some cases.

STAPHYLÆDEMA.—Relaxation of the Uvula. In some cases it is so tumefied and elongated as to occasion cough and difficulty in swallowing. It is always connected with a morbid condition of the stomach, and erythematic inflammation or "canker" of the mucous membrane of the throat. The local affection requires cold-water gargles and ice. If these do not reduce the uvula to comfortable dimensions, in due time, a portion of it—one-third to one-half—should be clipped off.

STAPHYLOMA.—Various tumors of the anterior surface of the globe of the eye have received this appellation.

STEARRHŒA.—Sebaceous Flux. Inordinate excretion from the sebaceous follicles of the skin, probably because the dietary is too hydro-carbonaceous, or greasy.

STEATOCELE.—Fatty Tumor of the Scrotum.

STEATOMA.—An encysted tumor whose contents are similar to fat. It should be removed with the knife.

STENIA.—Sthenia.

STERILITY.—Infecundity, Barrenness. It may depend on malformation of the genital organs. The most frequent cause is *dysmenorrhœa*. Leucorrhœa, with great relaxation of the os uteri, and menorrhagia, are sometimes the causes. "Irrespondence," or the absence of the sexual orgasm, on the part of the female, has been, though very erroneously, placed among the causes of sterility. Another cause may sometimes be found in constitutional infirmity, the female being incapable of developing a fully matured ovum. The medication must be directed to the removal of the cause, whatever that may be.

STERNALGIA.—Angina Pectoris.

STERNUTATION.—Sneezing. Sternutatory medicines—sneezing snuffs—constitute a class in the drugopathic materia medica; but such medication ought to be *sneezed* out of existence.

STERTOR.—Ronchus.

STHENIA.—Entony. The Entonic Diathesis; Inflammatory or Dynamic Fever. DUNGLISON's Medical Dictionary defines this, "Excess of strength;" but as such a condition is impossible, as much as is excess of health, or excess of truth, or excess of honesty, he must mean something else. The term only properly applies to phlegmonous inflammation and entonic fever, and means determination of morbid action to the whole surface of the body.

STILLICIDIUM.—Voiding urine only in drops.

STIMULATION.—This is said to be "the action of stimulants." But never was there a more egregious error—an error which is the parent source of all the dissipation and debauchery in the world. What is called *stimulus* or *stimulation*, so far from being the action of a dead, inert, inorganic matter on a living organism, it is a state of feverishness, irritation or inflammation; this being the action of the vital powers in resisting or expelling the poison. To stimulate a living organism is to

Stimulants are called *diffusible* or *permanent*, as they are supposed to act transiently, or to maintain their action persistently. But the rationale is, the vital powers act very vigorously in determining certain agents toward the cutaneous emunctory, while they resist others with less energy, and for that very reason, for a longer period, in the same direction. These are called *tonics*. When the rationale of stimulation is understood, there will be an end of *alcoholic* medication; and then, and not till then, will be hope for the temperance cause. For the full discussion of this subject, I must refer the reader to my recent work, "The True Temperance Platform."

STOMACACE.—Stomalgia; Cancer Oris, Canker, Cancer Aquaticus. Fetor of the mouth, with a bloody discharge from the gums. The term is also applied to scurvy.

STOMACALGIA.—Cardialgia.

STOMACHIC.—Medical dictionaries define this word, "A medicine which *gives* tone to the stomach." Unfortunately there is no such medicine. All the medicinal stomachics thus far discovered only *abstract* tone from the stomach.

STOMATITIS.—Inflammation of the mouth. If nothing injurious is taken into the mouth, the disease will, in due time, disappear.

STOMATITIS, APTHOUS.—See Apthæ.

STOMATITIS, MERCURIAL.—See Salivation.

STOMATITIS, OF NURSING WOMEN.—See Apthæ.

STOMATITIS, PSEUDO-MEMBRANEOUS.—Diptheritic Inflammation of the Mouth.

STOMATORRHAGIA.—Hemorrhage from the mouth. *Methodus medendi*—ice.

STONE IN THE BLADDER.—Vesical Calculi. By avoiding all impurities in the food and drink, almost all forms of calculous concretions in the bladder may be, in time, dissolved, and washed away. Whenever soft water is substituted for hard, these affections diminish.

STRABISMUS.—Squinting, Goggle-Eye. Discordance or disorder of the optical axes It is commonly dependent on inequality of the action of the motor muscles, or on a spasmodic condition of one of them. In some cases it is caused by inflammation of the brain, as in *Hydrocephalus Internus;* and occasionally it is owing to a difference of sensibility or irritability in the two eyes. When dependent on inequality or abnormal contraction of the muscle, it may be relieved by dividing the muscle at fault. In other cases it may be remedied by medicating the malady of which it is symptomatic.

STRAIN.—See Sprain.

STRANGERS' FEVER.—See Fever, Strangers'.

STRANGULATION.—Constriction, Suffocation. The compression of a part so as to seriously impede its circulation. It applies to hernial protrusions, hanging, choking, etc. When the protruded intestine is strangulated, as most frequently happens in *Inguinal Hernia*, efforts should be made immediately to reduce it, by the application of cold, and by manipulations with the hand. The process is sometimes greatly accelerated by having the patient's head downward, the hips resting against the side of a bed, or whatever else is convenient. If these measures fail, the only remedy is a surgical operation, which consists in carefully dissecting down to the part, and dividing the constricting fibers. The preventive remedy is a properly adjusted truss.

STRANGURY.—Dysuria. Extreme difficulty in voiding the urine, which only passes in drops. See Ischuria and Retention.

STREPITOSUS MORBUS.—Noisy Disease; a species of flatulence.

STRICTURE.—A diminution or contracted condition of some tube or duct. It most commonly affects the urethra, rectum, or œsophagus. They may be caused by a spasmodic contraction of the muscular fibers, or by a thickening of the mucous or lining membrane. In a majority of cases, they are connected with an inflammatory condition of the part, and will disappear when that is removed. In other cases the dilating gies must be resorted to. *Urethral stricture*, which is the most common and most distressing of all, is almost always the consequence of astringent or irritating injections, as lead, zinc, copper, corrosive sublimate, etc., which have been administered for the cure of gonorrhœa or nocturnal emissions. In treating several scores of cases, I have not met with one that resulted from any other cause.

STROKE, APOPLECTIC.—The occurrence of apoplexy.

STROKE, PARALYTIC.—Sudden occurrence of cerebro-spinal paralysis.

STROPHULUS.—Red-Gum, Tooth-Rash, White-Gum, Milk-Spots, Red-Gown. An eruption of red or whitish pimples, occurring in early infancy, chiefly about the face, neck, and arms. They exhibit much variety in appearance, are of no great importance, and only require the tepid ablution occasionally, with a little closer attention to fresh air, equable temperature, and simple diet.

STRUMA.—Scrofula.

STUFFING.—Cynanche Trachealis.

STUNNED.—Unconscious from a blow or fall. It was formerly the prevalent practice to bleed in this case, to "start the circulation." But, fortunately, the practice is now condemned as worse than useless, by the most eminent American and European physicians and surgeons. Pure air and perfect quiet are the best remedies.

STUPOR.—Diminished manifestation of the mental powers. There are all degrees, from partial lethargy to complete narcosis. The immediate cause is congestion of the brain; the remote causes are, excessive cold or heat, mental shock, narcotic drugs, etc. The treatment is the same as for apoplexy

STUTTERING.—See Stammering.

STYAN, STYE.—See Hordeolum.

STYPSIS.—Astriction, Constipation.

SUBLUXATION.—Sprain.

Submersion.—Drowning. Asphyxia by submersion is not owing to the introduction of water into the windpipe, as is commonly supposed, but to the non-introduction of atmospheric air; the spasmodic closure of the glottis prevents the water from entering the air passages until the exhaustion of the vital powers. See Asphyxia.

Subsultio.—Palpitation.

Subsultus Tendinum.—Clonus Subsultus, Saltus Tendinum, *Twitching of the Tendons.* Involuntary, instantaneous, and spasmodic contraction of the muscular fibres, communicating a jerking motion to the tendons. It is an indication of great irritation or exhaustion, and is generally noticed prominently in low and malignant fevers.

Succubus.—Nightmare; also a male or female phantom which appears to the opposite sex during lascivious dreams.

Sudamina.—Hydroata, Planta noctis. A miliary eruptive. See Miliary Fever.

Sudor.—Sweat, Miliary Fever.

Sudor Anglicus.—Sweating Fever, Sweating Sickness. This term has been applied to a severe epidemic disease which prevailed extensively in England and other parts of Europe, in the fourteenth, fifteenth, and sixteenth centuries, characterized by profuse sweating, with coldness, great prostration, and usually terminated, favorably or unfavorably, within twenty-four hours. It was very fatal, and was no doubt a malignant form of Miliary Fever.

Sudor Cruentus.—Cutaneous Hemorrhage, Bloody Sweat. Cutaneous perspiration mixed with blood.

Suffocation.—Strangling. See Asphyxia.

Suggillation.—A Bruise, Ecchymosis.

Summer Complaint.—A popular phrase including cholera, diarrhœa, and dysentery, and, indeed, all affections of the alimentary canal attended with vomiting or purging, or both. They are also termed "Summer Diseases." Deaths of these diseases constitute a large percentage of the mortality of our cities during the months of July and August, especially among children. Hot weather, unripe fruits, crude vegetables, and ill-ventilated apartments are among the causes of this "murdering of the innocents;" but the ordinary feeding and drugging of American children, is a tenfold greater cause of the "Infanticide." Tepid ablutions, cool wet cloths to the abdomen, abundance of fresh air, and good ripe fruit, are the essentials of the treatment. When bowel complaints prevail among children, the milk on which they are fed should be carefully looked to. An immense amount of "swill milk" is sold in our cities, and not a little in the rural districts, under the name of the "pure country" article. But, as rich men own the distilleries, and find it profitable to sell their alcoholized slops for "baby food," and as legislators and municipal officers are supposed to be susceptible to certain influences not here to be named, I see no chance for abating the evil, though the children are sent graveward in droves, until the people can receive a health education.

SUNBURN.—Rash, Freckle.

SUN-STROKE.—See *Coup de Soleil.*

SUPPRESSION.—Usually applied to amenorrhœa, but sometimes also to ischuria.

SUPPURATION.—Purulency; Formation of Pus. It may take place in any of the tissues. It is characterized by slight chills; remission of the lancinating pain, which becomes heavy; a sense of weight in the part, and when the part can be felt by fluctuation. When found on the surface, exposed to air, the part is called an ulcer, otherwise an abscess.

SURFEIT.—Colica Ciburia. See Colic, of Surfeit.

SUSPIRIUM.—Sigh, Suspiration, Short-Breathing.

SWEATING SICKNESS.—Miliary Fever. See Sudamia.

SWELLING.—Any abnormal increase of bulk. See Tumor.

SWELLING, WHITE.—See Hydrarthrus.

SWOON, SWOONING.—See Syncope.

SYCOMA, SYCOSIS.—See Ficus.

SYMPLEPHAROSIS. — Preternatural adhesion between the eye-lids.

SYMMETRICAL DISEASES. — A strange technicality, the offspring of a queer hypothesis. "It has been affirmed to be a law of the animal economy that, when uninfluenced by disturbing agents, all general or constitutional diseases affect equally and similarly the corresponding parts of the two sides of the body." This has been called, the *Symmetry of Disease;* and the resulting diseases are said to be *symmetrical.* A more rational "law of the animal economy," may be thus stated : when the whole mass of blood is so impure, or when the morbific condition is so great that all the vital powers are involved in the remedial struggle, as in the febrile diseases, the manifestations or phenomena of disease must necessarily be equal and similar in the corresponding parts of the two sides of the body.

SYMPTOSIS. — Depression, Emaciation, Collapse.

SYNANCHE. — Cynanche.

SYNCLONUS. — Tremulous agitation of various muscles.

SYNCOPE. — Fainting, Swoon. Complete and sudden loss of sensation and motion. The patient should be placed in the horizontal posture, and fanned or exposed to the fresh air. Sprinkling cold water over the face accelerates the recovery.

SYNECHIA. — Adhesion between the iris and transparent cornea, or between the iris and crystalline lens.

SYNEZISIS. — Occlusion or obliteration of the pupil. It may sometimes be remedied by the operation for artificial pupil.

SYNOCHA. — Cauma, Dynamic Fever, Entonic Diathesis, General Inflammation. See Fever, Inflammatory.

SYNOCHUS. — Mixed Fever, Synochoid; Common Continued Fever. This is defined to be, "continued fever compounded of inflammatory and typhus." The error consists in mistaking a mild form of putrid typhus for one kind of fever in the outset, and another in its progress. It is often termed "bilious fever with typhoid symptoms," or "synocha in the beginning, and typhus in the end."

SYNOVITIS.—Inflammation of the Synovial Membrane. It most frequently affects the knee-joint, and is a very obstinate malady. It is characterized by more or less heat, pain, and swelling, all of which are increased by standing or walking. Mercurial infection is the most common cause. It requires a persevering application of leg-baths, foot-baths, the wet-compress, and such general bathing as the state of the system calls for. The Hydro-Electrical bath is especially serviceable in these cases.

SYPHILIDES.—This term is applied to cutaneous eruptions which accompany syphilis. They are, in a great majority of cases, the effects of mercurial medicines.

SYPHILIS.—Lues Venera, Pox, French Pox. This form of venereal disease first appears in the form of *chancres*, or infectious ulcers, on the genital organs; if these are aggravated by improper treatment, or allowed to exist for many days, there will be more or less feverishness, with swelling and inflammation of the glands of the groin, called *bubo*, generally progressing to suppuration. The absorption of the virus eventually occasions ulcers in the throat, and copper-colored blotches on the skin, which are termed, *constitutional syphilis*. And when the patient is affected with pains in the bones, nodes, etc., these symptoms are termed, *tertiary syphilis*. But a long course of observation, and much experience in the treatment of syphilis, in all its forms and phases, primary and secondary, have satisfied me, beyond all shadow of doubt, that "constitutional" and "tertiary" syphilis are, in a very great majority of cases, the effects of mineral drugs, and not of the venereal disease. I have not, in a single case, known any secondary nor tertiary complications—no ulcers of the throat, no caries of the bones, no decomposition of the palate, no destruction of the nose, no nodes, etc., etc.—in patients whom I have treated for the primary symptoms, or who have not taken mineral medicines; and I have watched this point for more than twenty years. (A full account of syphilization and mercurialization may be found in my work, "Pathology of the Reproductive Organs.") The consequences of drug medication generally, and of mercurial "specifics" particularly, in all forms of venereal disease, are most horrible. The disease is bad enough; but the ordinary treatment is much worse.

The chancre should be thoroughly destroyed on its first appearance; aquafortis, nitrate of silver, or a red hot iron, may be employed for this purpose. One, two, three, or more applications may be required. The whole surface of the sore should be trouched every day, or every other day, until all appearance of virus or corrosion disappears, and healthy granulations appear at every point. If this treatment is promptly and properly pursued, and the patient subjected to a warm bath, or a wet-sheet pack daily, with a very abstemious and simple dietary, there will be no danger of buboes, nor of secondary, constitutional, nor tertiary symptoms.

Syphiloid.—Resembling Syphilis; Mercurial Cachexy.

Syspasia.—Clonic Spasm.

Tabes.—Marasmus. General emaciation.

Tabes Dorsalis.—Wasting of the body from sexual abuse.

Tabes Mesenterica.—Mesenteric Disease, Infantile Atrophy. Emaciation and wasting of the body with engorgement and tubercular degeneration of the mesenteric glands. It is one of the manifestations of the scrofulous diathesis.

Tænia.—Tape Worm. Only two species of intestinal worms, of the genus *Tenia*, are found in the human body, the *Tænia lata*, and *Tænia solium*. The former species is called the *Broad Tape Worm*, which has been known to reach sixty yards in length; the latter is known as the *Long Tape Worm*, and cases are recorded in which they attained the enormous length of six hundred feet. Many nostrums have acquired celebrity for destroying this species of worm—turpentine, male fern, pumpkin seed, etc.; but, like other worms which infest the bowels, they will disappear when the cause of their presence is removed. Probably none of them could long survive a

12

physiological dietary. They are by nature scavengers, as are flies, vultures, hogs and cockroaches; and when there is no appropriate food for them to subsist upon, they will necessarily die or *emigrate.*

TALIPES.—Club-Foot.

TALPA.—A tumor on the head, which has been supposed to burrow like a mole.

TARANTISMUS. — Tarantism, Tarentalismus, Chorea Sancti Valentini. A spasmodic affection in which the patients manifest an inordinate propensity to dance to the sound of music. No doubt the malady is frequently feigned. It was one of the epidemics of the middle-ages.

TEMULENTIA.—Inebriation, Drunkenness, Intoxication.

TENESMUS.—Frequent, painful, and vain desires to go to stool. It is a symptom in dysentery, and in piles.

TENIA.—Tænia.

TERTIAN FEVER.—Tertian Ague. Third day Intermittent.

TETANUS. — Constrictive Spasm. It is characterized by closure of the jaws; difficult deglutition, and rigidity of the limbs and trunk. When the spasm is confined to the muscles of the jaws, it is called *Trismus.* The body may be curved forwards, backwards, or to one side, constituting the forms termed *Emprosthotonos, Opisthotonos,* and *Pleurothotonos.* The immediate cause is generally the wounding of a nerve or tendon; sometimes mental shocks, or extreme exposures will occasion it. Certain narcotic drugs, *Strychnine, Bincine,* etc., in large doses, induce tetanic spasms.

The prolonged warm or tepid bath, or the hot-bath, followed by the tepid ablution, or dripping sheet, is our principal reliance in the treatment. In cases where the external temperature is considerably above the normal standard, constituting a general feverish condition, the wet-sheet pack is the preferable appliance. The patient should be kept as quietly as possible, and all sources of irritation removed as far as practicable

The ordinary remedy for tetanus, according to the "heal art," as it is in druggery, are, (I quote DUNGLISON's Dictionary, "Copious, and repeated blood-letting; bathing, cold and warm, powerful doses of opium, and other narcotics." If any one should, perchance, survive such treatment, it would be a powerful demonstration that *humanity is tough!*

TETTER.—See Herpes.

THELITIS.—Inflammation of the Nipple.

THEOMANIA.—Demonomania.

THERIOMA.—Any Malignant Ulcer.

THIRST, MORBID.—A symptom in many diseases. Nine-tenths of the thirst of the majority of persons, who call themselves well, is abnormal, and occasioned by unwholesome articles or preparations of food, condiments, irritants, etc.

THORACODYNE.—Pleurodynia. See Pleuralgia.

THORACYSTIS.—Hydatids of the Chest. Encysted Hydro-thorax.

THROAT-AIL.—Follicular Inflammation of the Fauces. It is always an indication of a morbid stomach or diseased liver, and can only be permanently cured by restoring the integrity of the digestive organs.

THROBBING.—Pain which is augmented by the arterial pulsations. This term is also applied to the strong, jerking motion of the heart or arteries.

THROMBUS.—Hæmatoma. A small, round, bluish tumor, formed by an effusion of blood into the areolar texture, in the vicinity of the vein which has been opened in the operation of venesection. It is commonly owing to the incision through the skin not corresponding exactly with that in the vein. Cold applications are proper.

THYMION.—A small wart, resembling a bud of thyme.

THYMIOSIS.—Frambœsia.

THYROCELE.—Bronchocele.

TIC.—Vellication, Twiching; habitual convulsive motion of certain muscles.

TIC DOULOUREUX.—Tic Douloureux, Neuralgia.

TINEA.—Porrigo.

TINNITUS AURIUM.—An imaginary sound, like that of the motion of the wind, the murmur of water, the ringing of a bell, etc. It often accompanies cerebral congestion, irritation.

TIXES.—Milk Sickness.

TITUBUTIO.—Fidgets.

TOBACCO-USING.—An extensive and rapidly increasing habit, and more ruinous to the human race than is the use of alcoholic beverages. It comprehends *chewing, snuffing, smoking,* and *dipping.* Tobacco-using, in all its forms, is the most filthy, indecent and disgusting habit to which depraved human nature was ever addicted. Those who would be relieved of this infernal infirmity, can mitigate the horrors of the transition state to purity and normal sensations, by taking a warm bath daily; adopting a very plain and abstemious diet; exercising very moderately; lying down whenever headache, restlessness, morbid irritability, mania, or *delirium tremens* become insupportable, and abstinence from all care or business, for a few days. Substitutes had better be let alone, as they only prolong the struggle, and may occasion a relapse.

TONIC SPASM.—Rigid contraction of the muscles without relaxation, as in tetanus.

TONICITY.—DUNGLISON defines this word: "The faculty that determines the general tone of the solids;" and he adds, "excessive tonicity causes *erethism* or *crispness;* deficient tonicity, *atony* or *weakness*." How can there be "excessive *faculty*" to determine tone? The author has made a distinction where there is no difference. Tonicity is not a faculty, for faculties are intellectual qualities; and it can no more be excessive than vitality or health can be excessive. "Erethism" of a part is simply disproportionate morbid action; and erethism of the whole system is simply preternatural determination of action to the whole surface; in other words, *entonic diathesis.* The error I am refuting is the cause of an incalculable amount of bleeding, antimonializing, depleting, and reducing practice, and occasions more deaths than "war, pestilence, and famine combined." To remedy erethism, or "excessive tonicity," we should not destroy the vitality, but balance the remedial action—a rule, by the way, which applies to all diseases; which has no exceptions, and which is absolutely infallible. And he is the most skillful physician, whether learned or illiterate in the technicalities of the medical profession, who best adapts his remedial appliances to this rule, in view of all the circumstances of the patient's case.

TONSILLITIS.—Inflammation of the Tonsils. See Quinsy.

TOOTHACHE.—See Odontalgia.

TOPHUS.—Calcareous concretions around the joints of gouty persons.

TORMENTUM.—Ileus; Intussusception. See Colic.

TORMINA.—Acute Colicky Pains.; Dysentery.

TORPID.—Inactive, Numb.

TORPOR, TORPITUDE.—Narcosis; Insensibility.

TORTICOLLIS.—Stiff-neck, Wry-neck. A rheumatic affection of the muscles of the neck, which inclines the head to the side. Fomentations will relieve all ordinary cases. If the muscles are permanently contracted, the remedy consists in dividing them.

TOXICAL.—Poisonous. The whole drug materia medica is but a collection of poisons; and their effects, though termed, "physiological," in medical books, are actually *toxicological*. If pharmacy was called *the art of mingling poisons*, as it truly is; and if drug medication was entitled, *the practice of poisoning the people, because they are sick*, as it really is, nobody would have anything to do with it.

TOXICOSIS.—Drug Diseases.

TRACHEITIS.—Cynanche Trachealis.

TRACHELISMUS.—Spasm of the Muscles of the Neck.

TRACHELITIS.—Cynanche Trachealis.

TRACHEOCELE.—Broncheocele.

TRACHEOPHTHISIS.—Laryngeal Consumption.

TRACHITIS.—Cynancho Trachealis.

TRACHOMA.—Granular Eyelid.

TRANCE.—Catalepsy, Ecstasis.

TRANSLATION OF DISEASE.—See Metastasis.

TRANSPLANTATION OF DISEASE.—PARACELSUS pretended to cure diseases by *transplantation*, which consisted in making them pass from one individual to another, either animal or vegetable. The pretension, though very absurd, is perfectly consistent with the theory which the *regular* physicians of the present day teach, concerning the nature of disease. If disease be really an entity, a thing, a substance, a something which "attacks us," "runs a course," "passes through us," "supervenes," "changes its seat," etc., etc., why could it not be driven out of the system? And if it can be driven *out* of one individual, what is to hinder it being driven *into* another?

TRANSPORT.—Delirium.

TREMBLES.—Milk Sickness.

TREMBLING.—Tremor.

TREMOR.— Trepidation, Trembling, Synclonic Spasm ; involuntary agitation of some one or all of the muscles. This disease is always connected with great debility or exhaustion, and is often occasioned by narcotic or mineral drugs. Hard drinkers, and workers in mercury, lead, etc., are very liable to it. These considerations sufficiently suggest the remedial plan.

TRICHIA.—Entropion.

TRICHIASIS.—Trichiosis. This term is applied to catarrh of the bladder, to inflammation of the breast, and to inversion of the eye-lashes.

TRICHINA SPIRALIS.—A small species of *entozoa*, discovered in the voluntary muscles. They are similar to the *eels* found in paste and vinegar. They are occasionally communicated to the human being through the beef, mutton, etc., on which he feeds.

Trichocephalus.—Long Thread-Worm. It generally inhabits the large intestines, especially the cæcum and colon. A physiological dietary is the remedy.

Trichosis.—Morbid condition of the Hair.

Trismus.—Partial Tetanus; Locked-Jaw.

Tromania.—Delirium Tremens.

Trumbus.—Thrombus.

Tubercule.—A tumor in the substance of an organ, from the production of new matter. Tubercles may form in any part of the body, but most frequently occur in the lungs and mesentery.

Tumor.—Swelling.

Turgescence.—Turgidity, Fullness, Congestion.

Turn of Life.—The cessation of the function of ovulation.

Tussis.—Tussicula, Cough, Bex. It is symptomatic of many diseases.

Tympanites.—Wind-Dropsy. Swelling of the abdomen from air accumulated in the peritoneum, or in the intestines. The abdomen sounds like a drum, when struck. It may be owing to exhalation of gas from the inner coat of the intestinal tube, or to decomposition of substances contained in it. It is always a dangerous symptom. When it occurs in low fevers after free bleeding, drastic purging, or severe drugging of any kind, it is almost invariably the precursor of death. The treatment consists in hot fomentations, or cold wet cloths, as the temperature of the part is below or above the normal standard. The heat may be variable, requiring corresponding alternations in the treatment. An enema of tepid water is proper, when there is evidence of fecal accumulation in the bowels.

Tympanitis.—This term is applied to inflammation of the lining membrane of the middle ear, and also to Tympanites.

Type.—The form of disease as relates to the periodicity of the paroxysms. It properly applies only to the febrile diseases, of which there are three types, *Continued, Remittent,* and

Intermittent. The term is used loosely, and in several senses, in medical writings. Thus, we read of dysentery of a malignant *type;* small-pox of a mild type; fever of the typhoid type, etc. There may be mild or malignant, typhoid or inflammatory, bilious or epidemic *forms* of disease, but there are no such types.

TYPHOID.—Resembling Typhus. The term typhoid is applied generically to all continued fevers of low or *atonic diathesis,* in contradistinction to inflammatory fever, which is *entonic diathesis.* It applies also to all visceral inflammations of the atonic diathesis. As the term is applied in medical writings to fevers, it generally means *nervous continued fever,* or the nervous form of typhus, in contradistinction to *putrid nervous fever,* or putrid form of typhus. The notion that typhoid fever is symptomatic of, or essentially connected with inflammation of PEYER's gland, while *typhus* is symptomatic of, or essentially connected with inflammation of BRUNNERS' gland, is one of the fallacies and fantasies that abound in medical books. Inflammation, and also ulceration of those glands may exist; not as a cause, however, but as an *effect* of the disease. See Fever, Nervous.

TYPHOMANIA.—The Delirium of Typhus or Typhoid Fever.

TYPHUS.—This term is usually applied to what I explain as *putrid continued fever.* It comprehends all continued fevers whose leading characteristic are grossness of the body, and impurity of the blood, as manifested in a dark coat of the tongue, foul breath, fetid excretions, crimson surface, blotches, spots, petechiæ, carbuncles, etc. Hospital, Jail, Ship, Camp, Spotted, Yellow, etc., fevers, and also plague, are forms of typhus. The terms, *Adynamic* and *Asthenic,* have been applied indiscriminately to both the nervous and putrid forms of fever; but more especially to those of the continued type. The "*rose* spots" and "mulberry rash" which some authors regard as peculiar to typhus, are not always present. They merely indicate a more severe or aggravated form of the disease. See Fever, Putrid.

ULATROPHIA.—Falling away of the Gums.

ULCER.—A Sore. Ulcers are variously divided into simple, sinuous, fistulous, fungous, gangrenous, scorbutic, syphilitic, cancerous, scrofulous, phagedenic, virulent, carious, varicose, indolent, erosive, etc. They are always symptomatic, and, hence, in their treatment the constitutional cause must be primarily regarded. The local treatment consists in regulating the temperature of the part, keeping it excluded as much as possible from the contact of air, by covering the surface or filling the cavity with fine flour, chalk-powder, or other absorbent and inert material, covering with simple cerate or adhesive plaster, and removing fungous granulations, callous edges, or adventitious formations, with caustic.

ULITIS.—Inflammation of the Gums.

URÆMIA.—A Urinous state of the Blood.

URETERALGIA.—Pain in the course of the Ureter. Calculus is the common cause.

URETERITIS.—Inflammation of the Ureter. It is commonly caused by calculus.

URETHRALGIA.—Pain in the Urethra.

URETHRITIS.—Gonorrhœa.

URETHROBLENORRHŒA.—Gonorrhœa, or Gleet.

URINE, INCONTINENCE OF.—See Eneuresis.

UROCRASIA.—Eneuresis.

URORRHŒA.—Eneuresis, Diabetis.

UROZEMIA.—Diabetis.

URTICARIA.—Nettle-Rash, Hives, Bold Hives. The eruption is distinguished by those elevations of the cuticle called *wheals*, and resembles that produced by the sting of the nettle. It is accompanied with intolerable itching, especially when the patient is warm in bed. It is of biliary origin, and is connected with gastric derangement. Tepid ablutions, and a plain, abstemious diet, will soon remove it.

UTEROMANIA.—Nymphomania.

UVULITIS.—Inflammation of the Uvula

12*

VACCINA.—Vaccinia, Cow-Pock, Kine-Pock, Inoculated Cow-Pox. The small-pox of the cow, called *cow-pox*, when transmitted to man, will, in most cases, protect him from the *small-pox*. Though medical authors are very fond of boasting of the discovery of JENNER, (whom the profession persecuted,) it has long been a controverted question whether his discovery of vaccina, as a preventive of small-pox, has been a blessing or a curse to the world. We are of opinion its evils immeasurably overbalance all the good the world has derived from it. There is something revolting to plain, unsophisticated common sense in the idea of *infecting* the blood of a healthy person with some bane or baleful thing, some venom or virus, to produce immunity from disease; yet it is in character with the whole drug system. And quite recently *syphilization* has been gravely proposed as a preventive of venereal disease! And why not? If persons ought to be poisoned, because they are sick, the same reasoning would poison and infect them to preserve health; and it does. The vaccine virus is usually taken from the human vesicle; but this exposes the innoculated person to a worse infection than that of small-pox. Scrofula and venereal disease are often communicated in this way. Vaccina requires no other treatment than a daily ablution, with due attention to the dietary.

Modified small-pox, termed *varioloid*, is the small-pox occurring after successful vaccination. It is sometimes epidemic.

VACCINATION.—This operation consists in inserting the vaccine virus under the cuticle, or scarf-skin, so that it may come in contact with the absorbents. The best time for taking the matter is about the eighth day, when it ought to be limpid and transparent. The scab, which falls off in about twenty days, is often employed; but it is less reliable.

VAGINITIS.—Inflammation of the Vagina. This term is often applied to leucorrhœa. This affection is not uncommon. and commonly not difficult to cure. But when aggravated with astringent and caustic injections, it often becomes exceedingly obstinate and distressing. Tepid, cool or cold injections, hip-baths, and the wet-girdle, are the special appliances.

Vagitus.—Squalling. The cry of the new-born child.

Varicella.—Chicken-Pox; Bastard Small-Pox. It is characterized by transparent vesicles, about the size of peas, scattered over the body. There are several varieties; some of which are called swine-pox, water-pox, water-jags, etc. It is an unimportant affection, and cleanliness is all that is necessary to regard in the matter of treatment.

Varicoblepharon.—Varicose Tumor of the Eyelid.

Varicocele.—Spermatocele, Cirsocele. Varicose dilatation of the veins of the scrotum and spermatic cord. It is a soft, knotty, compressible tumor, situate in the course of the cord, and increasing from below upwards. It does not usually cause much inconvenience, and a suspensory bandage is all the treatment necessary.

Variola.—Small-Pox. There are two forms of this disease, the *discreet*, or *distinct*, and the *confluent*. In the first named variety, the pustules are nearly the size of peas, distinct, distended, and circular, and the fever is *inflammatory*. In the confluent form the pustules are irregularly circumscribed, and run together, and the fever is *typhoid*. In the distinct or mild form, the pustules appear from the third to the fifth day, and suppurate from the eighth to the tenth. In the confluent or malignant form, the course of the symptoms are less uniform. The constitutional disturbance which precedes and accompanies the eruption is termed *Eruptive Fever*, and that which succeeds the pustules, and which occurs from the tenth to the thirteenth day, is termed the *Secondary Fever*.

Small-pox represents the most putrescent of the exanthems, or eruptive fevers, as the plague does the extreme of grossness and putrescency among the simple fevers; hence the prime importance of an abundance of fresh air, light, and a cool, equable temperature. The temperature of the apartment (and this rule applies with emphasis to all eruptive fevers, and with especial emphasis to small-pox,) should always be as low as the patient can bear, without absolute chilliness. The constitutional symptoms—the fever—should be treated precisely as all other fevers of the same type and diathesis. The external applications must be regulated by the temperature of the skin. The greater the morbid heat and dryness, the more frequently should it be bathed or sponged, and the cooler or colder should be the temperature of the water employed. When the diathesis of the fever is inflammatory, the wet-sheet pack daily is preferable; it is also to be preferred in the typhoid cases, except when the pulse is low, and there is a disposition to chilliness, or to coldness of the extremities. In these cases, tepid ablutions should be frequently employed. Pure water, of any temperature most agreeable to the patient, may be taken *ad libitum;* no food at all should be taken until the eruption on the surface is well established, and very little, and that only of mild, ripe, juicy fruits and gruel, until the process of pustulation is completed. To prevent pitting, cold wet cloths should be kept constantly on the parts exposed to the air, and the sores covered with fine flour, chalk-powder, or something to protect them from atmospheric air.

VARIOLOID.—Modified Small-Pox. This is small-pox occurring after vaccination. The matter of a varioloid pustule will occasion small-pox in one who has never had the disease "the natural way." Varioloid sometimes prevails epidemically, but is a much milder disease than variola. It requires no other attention than light diet and tepid ablutions.

VARIX.—Varicose Vein; Dilatation of a Vein. Varicose tumors occur most frequently in the superficial veins of the lower extremities, and are owing to relaxation or obstruction. They are soft, unequal, knotty, and livid. They will often disappear when the general tone of the muscular system is restored, or the particular cause of the obstruction, (as the pressure of the gravid uterus, an enlarged liver, extreme constipation, etc.,) are removed. In severe cases, they require to be checked by, and compressed with, an appropriate bandage. The radical cure, in bad cases, is by caustic or ligature.

VENOM.—A poisonous fluid, secreted by certain animals, as the viper, rattlesnake, etc.

VENOSITY.—An unusual preponderance of venous or impure blood. Whatever tends to obstruct the eliminating functions, especially those of the lungs and skin, favors the production of a carbonaceous or impure state of the whole mass of the blood. This condition is seen in dropsy, plethora, asphyxia, etc., and in low fevers of the putrid form. To cure venosity, it is only necessary to *arterialize* or purify the blood. And yet, strange as it may seem, the celebrated author, ROKITANSKY, who is said to be the greatest pathologist now living, teaches that consumption is owing *to a want of venosity* in the blood! or too great a proportion of pure blood!! And his treatment is consistent with his theory, and with the practice of our allopathic brethren all over the civilized world—hydro-carbonaceous diet, drink, and medicine, as pork, grease, cod-liver oil, alcohol, etc., etc.

VENTOSITY.—Flatulence.

VERMINOUS.—Caused by Worms. Many symptoms of obstruction, indigestion, and constipation in children are erroneously attributed to worms, and the patient drugged with pink, senna, turpentine, powdered glass, or calomel, which occasion more mischief, frequently in a single hour, than the worms would, if let alone, in a whole year.

VERRUCA.—Wart. A few touches of nitric acid, nitrate of silver, or any other strong caustic, will destroy them, as their vitality is very low, comparatively.

VERTIGO.—Giddiness, Dizziness, Swimming of the Head. In this condition the patient experiences sensations as if all objects were circumvirating around him. It is immediately owing to congestion of the brain, and often precedes apoplexy, epilepsy, etc.

VESANIA.—Madness.

VESICATION.—The formation of Blisters. The medical dictionaries say, "The action of a vesicant," but as vesicants do not act in the production of blisters, the definition is a failure. The practice of destroying some part of the surface, because another part is in a bad way, is of a piece with the philosophy of poisoning the whole body through and through, because it is sick.

VIBICES.—Spots. Large purple discolorations of the skin. which appear in malignant putrid fevers. They resemble the marks produced by the strokes of a whip, and indicate extreme putrescency.

VICARIOUS.—This term is applied to secretions, excretions, hemorrhages, and diseases, when they appear to be substitutes for, or to take the place of, some other affection or action. Thus, nose-bleeding at the menstrual period would be called vicarious hemorrhage; increased discharge of urine, because the action of the skin was diminished, would be called vicarious urination, etc. The practitioner should carefully watch the evidences of, and as far as possible obviate the necessity for, vicarious functional duty, without, however, directly repressing it, as is the ordinary practice.

VIGILANCE.—Insomnia.

VIRUS.—Prof. DUNGLISON defines this word, "the agent for the transmission of infectious diseases." It is the *cause* of infectious diseases, not the agent by which they are transmitted. It is the poison which, being resisted or expelled by the vital powers, occasions the disease we call infectious. Infection is unappreciable by any chemical or physical tests, and the result of a morbid process, thereby differing from *venom*, which is an ordinary excretion or secretion.

VIS MEDICATRIX NATURÆ.—This term is usually defined, "the inherent and instinctive healing power, in an animal or vegetable, by virtue of which it can repair injuries inflicted upon it, or remove disease." A world of delusion will be removed from the minds of medical men, when they can understand that, so far from the *vis medicatrix naturæ* being the power that removes the disease, *it is the disease itself*. And when the people recognise this great truth, they will demand a very different method of medicating their maladies, than that which has been in vogue for some three thousand years.

Vomica.—Collections of purulent matter in the lungs, which open into the bronchial tubes, and are discharged by the mouth, constituting the *apostematous* form of consumption. See Consumption, Apostematous.

Vomit, Black.—The vitiated matter ejected from the stomach in yellow fever and other putrid diseases.

Vomiting.—Spewing, Puking.   See Emesis.

Vomiturition.—Retching, Heaving, Ineffectual efforts to vomit.

Vulvitis.—See Vaginitis.

Wale.—Wheal.

Wart.—See Verruca.

Washerwoman's Scall.—A species of Psoriasis, which see.

Wasp, Sting of.—The poison may be decomposed by any caustic which will slightly disorganize the part to which it is applied, as aquafotis, aqua ammonia, or sulphate of zinc. The inflammation may be assuaged by means of very cold water or ice.

Waterbrash.—See Pyrosis.

Water-Jags.—See Varicella.

Water-Pox.—Varicella.

Water-Qualm.—Pyrosis.

Weaksightedness.—Asthenopia.

Weal.—Wheal.

Weaning Brash.—See Brash, Weaning.

Web-Eye.—Caligo.

Welk.—Whelk.

Wen.—Tumor. Indolent, circumscribed and non-inflammatory tumors, occuring in any part of the body, are termed *wens*. They sometimes increase to an enormous size. The remedy is extirpation with the knife.

Wheal.—Wale, Weal. Elevations or ridges of the skin, as if produced by a rod or whip. They are seen in urticaria.

WHELK.—Welk. See Gutta Rosea.

WHISKY LIVER.—See Liver, Nutmeg.

WHITE SWELLING.—See Hydrarthus, and Phlegmatia Dolens.

WHITES.—See Leucorrhœa.

WHITLOW.—See Paronychia.

WHOOPING COUGH.—See Pertussis.

WIND DROPSY.—Emphysema, Tympanites.

WINDINESS.—Flatulence.

WORMS.—Entozoa, Vermes. Animals which are known to exist only in other animals, are found not only in the natural cavities, but also in the tissue of the organs.

The following is a tabular arrangement of the entozoa, with their usual habitual, which have been found in the human body:

Entozoa.	Where found.
Trichocephalus dispar, Oxyuris vermicularis, Ascaris lumbricoides, Bothriocephalus latus, Tænia solium, Ditrachyceras rudis,	Intestines.
Diplosoma crenata, Spiroptera hominis, Dactylius aculeatus,	Urinary Bladder.
Distoma hepaticum,	Gall Bladder.
Strongylus gigas.	Kidney.
Filaria oculi,	Eye.
Echinococcus hominis,	Liver, Spleen, and Omentum.
Polystoma pinguicola,	Ovary.
Polystoma venarum seu sanguicola Hexathyridium venarum,	Veins.
Filaria bronchialis,	Bronchial Glands.
Trichina spiralis, Cysticercus cellulosæ,	Muscles.
Acephalocystis multifida,	Brain.
Filaria medinensis,	Cellular texture.

The most common of these are the Oxyures, Ascarides, and Tænia, which are found in the intestines. There are no symptoms which positively indicate their presence, except their discharge. As they are never found outside of a living organism, and only subsist within on the *offal* of the alimentary canal, being essentially scavengers, it is clear that a physiological dietary is the chief and probably all-sufficient remedy.

WOUND.—Mechanical Injury. Any sudden solution of continuity, or displacement of parts by some mechanical force. They are distinguished into incised, punctured, lacerated, and poisoned. Aside from the surgery, water dressings to regulate the temperature, or in other words, control the inflammation, are all the treatment which can be necessary or useful.

WRENCH.—Sprain.

WRIST-DROP.—Paralysis of the muscles of the forearm, occasioned by the poison of lead.

WRITER'S SPASM.—See Spasm, Writer's.

XANTHOPSIA.—Yellow Vision, Jaundice.

XANTHOSIS.—The yellow discoloration which is often observed in cancerous tumors.

XANTHURIA.—Depoits of xanthic oxide in the urine.

XEROPHTHALMIA.—Lippitudo, also an inflammation of the eye without discharge.

YAWNING.—Gaping. A deep, slow inspiration, followed by a prolonged and slightly sonorous expiration. It indicates torpor, or fatigue of the respiratory system, and is an effort to promote aeration of the blood.

YAWS.—See Framboesia.

YELLOW FEVER.—See Fever, Yellow.

YELLOWS.—Jaundice.

ZELOSIS, ZELOTYPIA.—Melancholy, Mania.

ZOANTHROPIA.—A species of monomania in which the sufferer imagins himself transformed into an animal.

ZOARA.—Insomnia.

APPENDIX.

HYGEIO-THERAPEUTIC MOVEMENTS.

As there are many cases of disease and infirmity for which it is impossible to give special directions, in a work of this kind, for such gymnastic, calisthenic, or kinesipathic exercises and manipulations as may be desirable in the course of treatment, I have deemed it important to supply, in an appendix, such instructions and illustrations as will enable those who cannot avail themselves of the advantages of teachers, nor the privileges of Health Institutions, in a measure to "work out their own salvation." I would, however, recommend to all who desire fuller instructions and a greater variety of illustrations than can be given here, to study the various works on this subject, particularly the author's "Illustrated Family Gymnasium," published by FOWLER & WELLS, No. 389 Broadway, New York.

GENERAL RULES.

The following remarks are copied from the above mentioned work, with the kind permission of the publishers:

"It is no doubt a correct maxim, that all violent exertions should be made when the stomach is empty, or nearly so. The best times for the most active gymnastic exercises are early in the morning and towards evening; when practiced at or near bedtime, they should be more moderate. They should never be practiced immediately after meals, nor very near the time for eating, as digestion is never well performed when the system is in an agitated, or exhausted condition.

"Exercises should always be commenced, as well as finished, gently. This is especially important for new beginners, as they are sometimes injured, and their progress retarded by too severe efforts at first. As a general rule, all very abrupt transitions are objectionable.

"Let the pupil never forget that the organs or parts are to be developed and strengthened by moderate and prolonged exertions, rather than by violent and fitful ones.. The weaker organs or limbs should always receive most attention, and be more frequently subjected to exercises specially adapted to their invigoration."

"The dress should always be light and easy, and all superfluities in the dress itself, or in the pockets, as toys, knives, etc., dispensed with. Pupils should be careful and not sit in

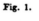

a draught of cold air, nor drink very much cold water, nor lie down on damp or cold ground when fatigued from exercise. Nor should they bathe or wash all over when much fatigued. A high temperature, perspiration, or 'feverishness' of the body, is, in itself, no objection to cold bathing, but rather an indication for it, provided the body is not at all fatigued, and the respiration is not disturbed."

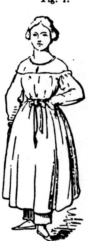

Exercising Dress.

"It is always important to vary the exercises frequently, so as to call into action alternately various sets of muscles. When large classes take lessons together, it is a good plan to divide them into sub-classes, giving the easier exercises to the smaller and weaker."

BODILY POSITIONS.

"In all kinds of gymnastic performances, as well as in all occupations, it is essential to observe undeviatingly, correct bodily positions. In lying, sitting, standing, walking, riding or laboring, the trunk of the body is to be kept erect. The bending is to be done on the hip-joint, and not by crooking the spinal column forward, and thus forcing the ribs and sternum in upon the stomach and lungs. Immense mischief results from this habit."

"Bolsters and high pillows are among the abominations of fashionable life. The head should never be raised more than a few inches, by a single *small* pillow. But it is a general custom to pile pillow on pillow, like 'Alps on Alps,' until the poor doubled and twisted victim is elevated out of all reasonable shape, and the neck so bent, and lungs so compressed, that congestion is sure to affect the brain, while free breathing is utterly impossible. Dullness of mental comprehension, and general torpor or stupidity of the intellectual faculties are among the consequences of this pernicious habit."

Fig. 2.

The military position, which brings the ear, shoulder, hip, knee and ankle into a line, is the proper standing position, as seen in fig. 2.

In this position the shoulders are squared, the heels placed slightly apart in line, the toes out to an angle of sixty degrees, the knees straight, the arms hanging easily by the side, and the hands open to the front. The chest must be slightly inclined forward, the abdomen moderately drawn in, the head erect, the eyes looking directly forward, and the weight of the body resting more on the fore

The Military Position. part of the feet than on the heels.

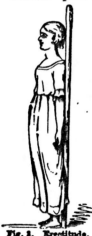

Fig. 3 represents an excellent position for straightening a crooked spine and securing erectitude of body, with free and unrestrained action of the whole respiratory system. It may be assumed in the standing and lying positions alternately, and, although it may prove difficult and painful to maintain this attitude at first, it will soon become easy. The person may stand against a wall, or lie on the floor, for a few minutes at a time, and repeat the exercises as many times a day as convenient.

Fig. 3. Erectitude.

ABDOMINAL MANIPULATIONS.

In many cases of dyspepsia, attended with a rigid or relaxed, and, consequently, feeble condition of the abdominal and dorsal muscles, spatting, kneading, thumping and rubbing, with the hand, are very useful, and often very important exercises. They should never be so violent nor prolonged as to occasion more than temporary pain or inconvenience. They should be performed for a few minutes while the patient lies on the back, and then with the patient lying face downward. As the muscles of the abdomen and back run in all directions—transverse, longitudinal and oblique—the rubbing motions should be correspondingly varied, so as to stir all of the muscles in the direction of their fibres. When kneading or spatting the abdomen or back, the patient should be directed to expand the lungs by a full inspiration, and to hold the breath as long as possible, while the "percussion" is being performed. For spinal irritations and curvatures, great benefit may be derived from gently, but perseveringly, spatting and rubbing the muscles along the spinal column for ten or fifteen minutes, daily. For habitual constipation, kneading the muscles of the abdomen is the specialty of "movement cure."

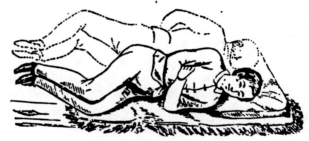

Fig. 4. Turning of the Body.

There are some movements which the patient can perform without an assistant or manipulator, which are admirably adapted to overcome torpor and sluggishness of the abdominal organs.

"With a mattress to lie upon, and a small pillow for the head, the patient lies down on the back, with the arms folded across the breast, the legs half bent at the knee, and the feet resting on the floor. The whole body then makes a simple turning motion which brings it on the arm, shoulder, and the side of the hip-joints, then back again, and then the same to the other side. The movement should be a complete change of the body from a back to a side position, so that it forms a semicircle."

The aim of the motion is not so much exercise of the muscles—for here there is no particular use of them, and the amount is unimportant, which is the reason that this movement has nothing straining or fatiguing—as a rocking, *alternating change of position of the more easily moved inner organs*, especially the *abdominal intestines*. Such a change of position may, however, be, in a simple manner, a means of causing many a cure, or at least of aiding in doing so, as every physician knows. So, for instance, for a more regular distribution of blood in all such cases where the *obstruction of the circulation of the blood in the organs of the lower part of the abdomen* requires remedy, as in cases of *hemorrhoidal tumors* (not yet inflamed, but already, perhaps, in an advanced state), of *contraction of the urinary bladder*, which stands in connection with the above; or *congestion of blood in the abdomen before the menstrual period of females*, giving cause to hemorrhage, etc. It is further of use in preventing or removing *flatulence*, also for the reduction of *strangulated hernia*.

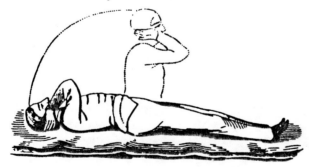

Fig. 5. Raising of the Trunk.

Raising of the trunk is another very useful and very convenient exercise. The body must be placed in a horizontal position, on a bed, mattress, or carpet; or two cushions, one under the head and the other under the hips, will answer all purposes. The exercise consists simply in raising the trunk to an upright position, without moving the legs. Many will require the assistance of a block of wood, or a heavy cushion, at first, which, being laid across the legs above the ankle, serves as a compensation weight. After a little practice, this may be dispensed with. At first the arms should be crossed over the breast. If this succeeds, the hands may then be placed behind the head, as in the illustration. If it is desirable to render the movement still more difficult, and put the muscles in greater tension, dumb-bells may be used, the hands being held close down by the body.

"This is a movement setting powerfully in motion all the muscles of the abdomen, but more especially those of the fore part, whose activity, and the straining they undergo, exert a direct and very decided influence on the functions of the body, but which are, however, just those that are in so

Fig. 6.

Combination Movement.

many cases so much neglected. After a repetition of the motion for a few times, the beneficial influence of it will be already experienced by the feeling of warmth which immediately follows, and spreads itself over the whole region of the abdomen."

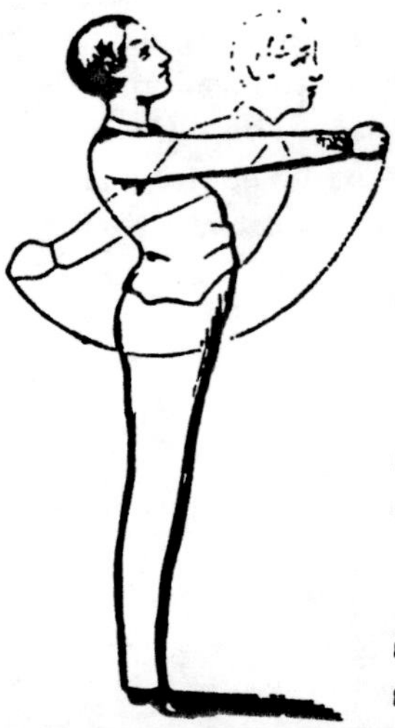

"For very feeble patients, and for female weaknesses, where the abdominal muscles are very much relaxed, the patient may have the head slightly raised. A sofa or lounge can be easily arranged for this purpose.

A combination movement, to act on the whole respiratory system, as well as the abdominal muscles, is represented in fig. 6. The arms are stretched out, but not stiffly, with the fists closed, and then thrown forcibly backward and forward.

The trunk must not remain stiff, but rather yielding upon the hip-joints, in such a manner that, acting as a balance, it is now bent a little forward, now a little backward, according as the arms are swinging backward or forward. The whole movement is thereby rendered easier, and the effect more universal. Besides the respective arm and shoulder muscles, most of those of the abdomen and back are set in a sort of rocking motion. The immediate effect of this motion is an agreeable feeling, and although the motion itself is somewhat violent, its influence is, on the whole, a mild one. It powerfully promotes a general and equable circulation of the blood, and is of essential benefit in cases of sub-paralysis or extreme torpor of the muscles of the arm, back, and abdomen, and is a most excellent preparatory exercise for a course of gymnastics. For sedentary persons, and for young persons with contracted chests and consumptive tendency, it cannot be too highly recommended.

THORACIC MOVEMENTS.

To expand the chest and enlarge the whole breathing apparatus, the Indian club exercises are excellent. The following remarkable instance of its beneficial effects is copied from the *Illustrated News:*

"We learn that Mr. HARRISON first began to use the clubs three years ago, at which time his muscular development was regarded as being very great; his measurement being then: Round the chest, thirty-seven and a half inches; round the upper arm, thirteen and seven-eighths inches, and round the forearm, thirteen and one-fourth inches. The clubs with which Mr. HARRISON commenced, weighed about seven pounds each; he has advanced progressively, until he can now wield with perfect ease two clubs, each weighing thirty-seven pounds, and his heaviest weighs forty-seven pounds. The effect of this exercise on the wielder's measurement is as follows: Round the chest forty-two and a half inches; the upper arm, fifteen inches, and the forearm fourteen inches. At the same time his shoulders have increased immensely,

13

and the muscles of his loins, which were weak when he first used the clubs, are now largely developed and powerful. In short, all the muscles of the trunk have been much improved by this exercise." The robust appearance of Mr. HARRISON

after three years' ex-
periment, is repre-
sented is fig. 7.

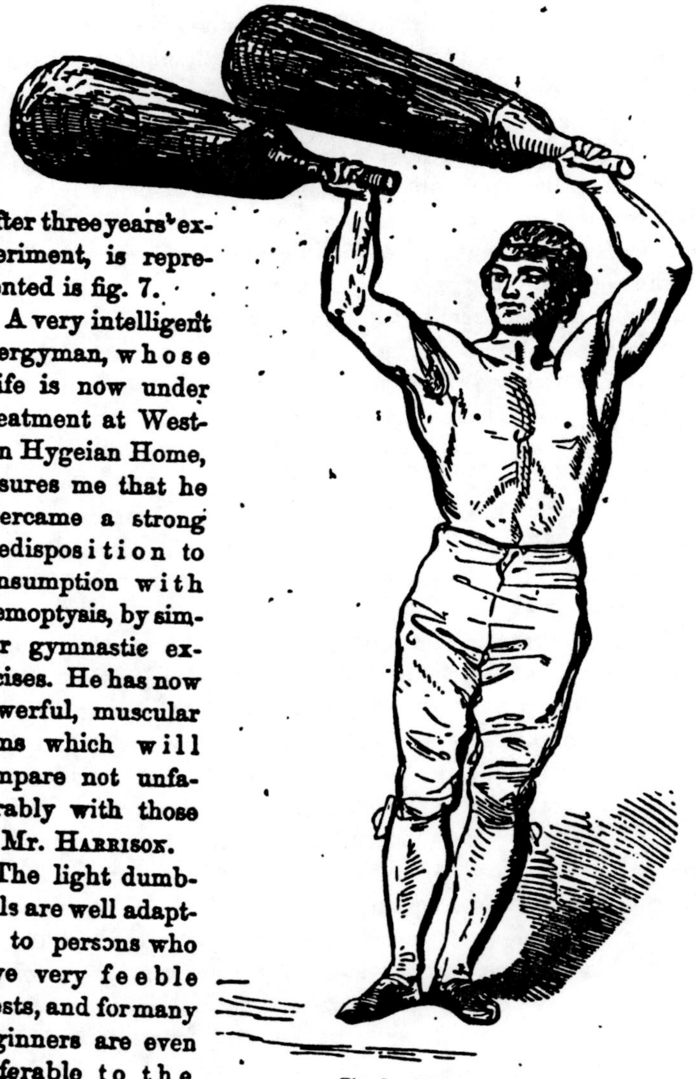

A very intelligent clergyman, w h o s e wife is now under treatment at West-ern Hygeian Home, assures me that he overcame a strong predisposition to consumption w i t h hæmoptysis, by sim-ilar gymnastic ex-ercises. He has now powerful, muscular arms which w i l l compare not unfa-vorably with those of Mr. HARRISON.

The light dumb-bells are well adapt-ed to persons who have very feeble chests, and for many beginners are even preferable to the

Fig. 7. Mr. Harrison.

clubs. Figs. 8 and 9 represent one of the many useful exercises which can be performed with them.

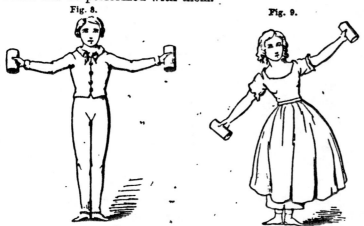

Fig. 8.   Fig. 9.

Exercises with the Dumb-Bells.

When the weights are extended horizontally, the pupil may advantageously march to counting or music.

FREE EXERCISES FOR SEDENTARY PERSONS.

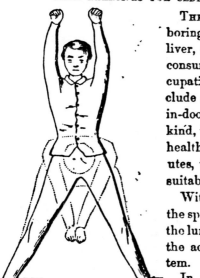

Fig. 10. Chopping Motion.

THERE are many persons laboring under dyspepsia, torpid liver, constipated bowels, and of consumptive tendency, whose oc cupations or circumstances preclude ordinary outdoor, or much in-door exercise of a healthful kind, who might keep up their health by devoting twenty minutes, twice a day, to gymnastics suitable to their condition.

With nearly all such persons the special indications are to keep the lungs expanded, and promote the action of the digestive system.

In addition to the exercises already pointed out, there are

few which may be very conveniently practiced by almost all persons of sedentary occupations, especially adapted to invigorate the respiratory and digestive organs, and, if duly attended to, would prove infallible as a preventive of that prevalent malady of our country, consumption.

In the first place, let the patient or gymnast purify the air in the lungs thoroughly, by, drawing in the abdominal muscles upon the diaphragm, throwing the chest forward, and expiring all the air out of the lungs possible; then inhale slowly till the lungs are filled to their utmost capacity, retain the whole volume of air in the lungs a few moments, and then expire or blow it out as completely as possible. This may be repeated from half a dozen to a dozen times, which will serve, in most cases, to decarbonize the lungs effectually.

Some persons, not accustomed to gymnastic respiratory movements, may experience, at first, some degree of vertigo or dizziness; but this will soon wear off. Such persons, should, however, be gentle in their first exercises.

Next, the movement represented in fig. 10, called the chopping motion, may be practiced a few minutes. The lungs should expire as the hands descend, and inspire as the body regains its erect posture, taking care to have the lungs fully

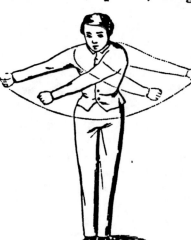

inflated each time the body becomes erect.

These movements act in one direction quite powerfully on the sluggish rectal and transverse muscles of the abdomen; and then, by resorting to the mowing movement, (fig. 11), we bring the action more directly on the oblique muscles and internal organs. After performing these motions a few times, they should be so extended as to bring the points of the

Fi 11. Mowing Motion.

fingers down to the floor on each side. The same precautions as to respiration are necessary here as in the preceding movement.

Fig. 12.

The sawing movement may next be practiced. One arm is thrown forward as the other is drawn back, precisely as though you were striking at an object with one hand, and drawing it toward you with the other. This produces a very general or universal action of the muscular system.

The joints of the lower extremities should lastly be specially brought into play, by a few of the rising and sinking movements, as shown in fig. 12.

The exercises may be concluded with any familiar dancing step, or with the

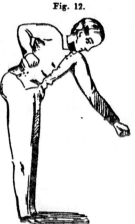

Sawing Movement.

trotting movement [fig. 14], which consists in hopping on the points of the toes, first with one foot, ten, twenty, fifty or one

Fig. 13. Fig. 14.

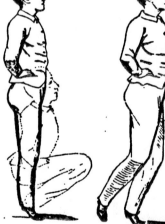
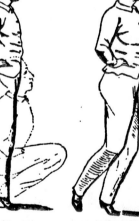

Flexion. Hop Movement.

hundred times, and then with the other. This movement may be easy or severe, as it is prolonged on one foot, and according to the height of the hop. In moderation, it is an excellent sleep-promoting and soothing exercise for nervous invalids.

PROMISCUOUS EXERCISES.

A variety of useful illustrations, which were selected and arranged for the *Water-Cure Journal* for 1853, are well adapted to individual cases and for family use, and may be properly introduced in this place.

In fig. 15, the feet being placed close, the hands fixed on the hips, rise on the toes, then bend the knees, and lower the body gradually till the thighs touch the heels; extend the arms in front, and fall forward, so that the body forms a straight line from the head to the heels, and rests on the hands and toes. These motions call into powerful action nearly three hundred muscles—those of the upper and lower extremities, chest, spine, and abdomen.

Fig. 15.

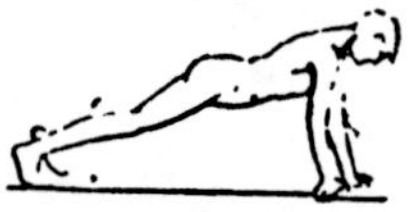

The action in fig. 16 is intended to exert mainly the muscles of the lower extremities alone. The feet being placed close, the hands open, the arms straight upward, the palms in front, bend the body forward, and touch the ground with the points of the fingers. The knees are to be kept straight.

Fig. 16.

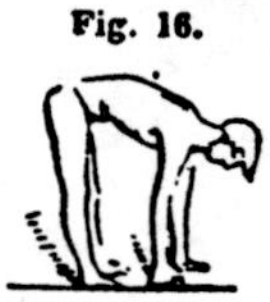

The exercise in fig. 17 acts particularly on the muscles of the toes, ankle-joints and hips. The feet close, the hands on the hips, cross the legs, bend the knees gradually, sit down, and rise again.

Fig. 17.

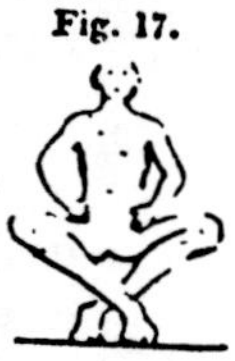

The action in fig. 18 throws the whole effort on the muscles of one of the lower extremities. The feet close, the arms extended in front, raise the left leg in front, bend the right knee gradually, and sit down on the ground, then get up again in the same position.

Fig. 18.

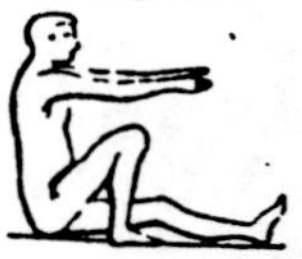

The action in fig. 19 is performed by two persons facing each other, so as to act upon the muscles of the upper and lower extremities simultaneously. The left hand on the hip, the right foot in front, lock the middle finger in each other's right hand, and pull backward.

Fig. 19.

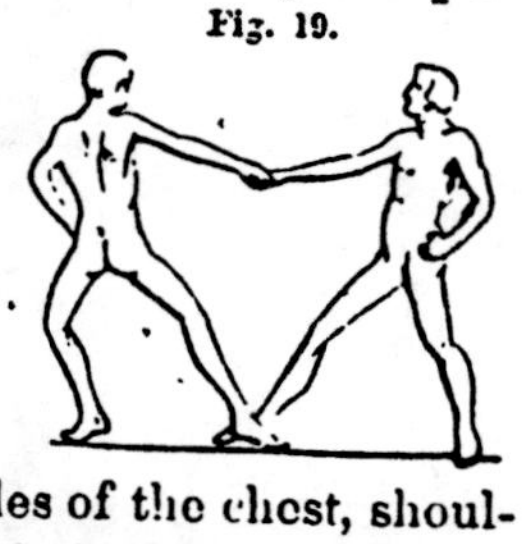

The action in fig. 20 brings into play the muscles of the chest, shoulders, and upper portion of the back. Let the palms of the hands touch behind, fingers pointing downward; turn the fingers inward, and bring the hands as high as possible up the back, taking care to keep the palms of the hands close together.

Fig. 20.

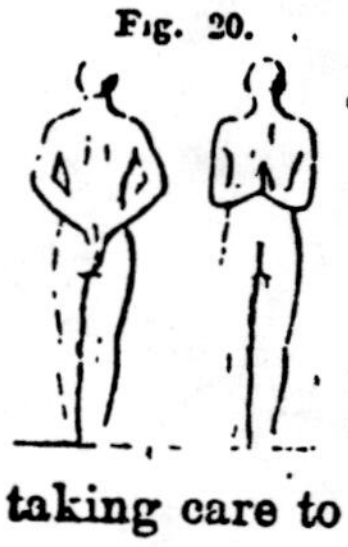

In fig. 21 the action is calculated to give great power and flexibility to the muscles of the legs and feet. The feet close, the hands on the hips, jump up and spread out the legs and close them alternately.

Fig. 21.

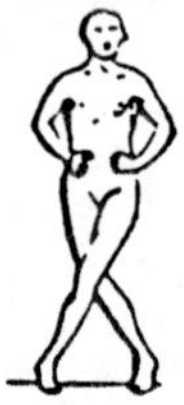

In fig. 22 the action is performed by two persons sitting down, who face each other, the soles of the feet touching, then grasping a stick and pulling against each other, first with knees straight, secondly with knees bent, and thirdly with the legs open. The principal force is exerted by the muscles of the arms, and those about the knee-joints.

Fig. 22.

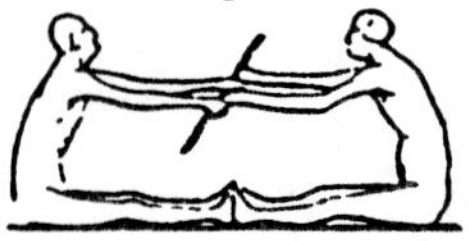

Fig. 23 mainly exerts the muscles of the toes and legs. The hands are placed on the hips, the right foot in front, the toe pointing downward; spring or jump twice on the right toe, and twice on the left, alternately, the knees being kept straight.

Fig. 23.

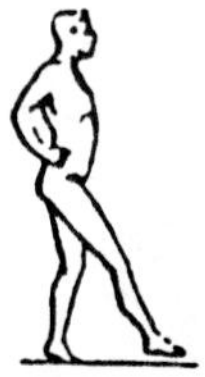

Fig. 24 exercises the muscles of the upper extremities, small of the back, and feet. In performing this exercise, take hold of each other's hands, with the toes opposite; then lean back and go round quickly.

Fig. 24.

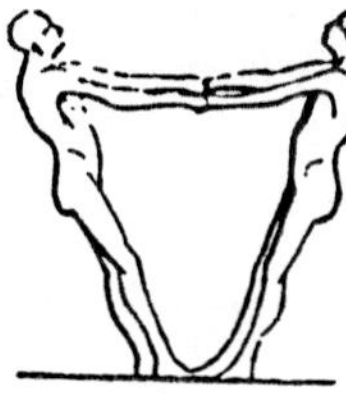

In fig. 25 the action exercises the pectoral muscles, with those around the shoulder joint. Grasp the left hand with the right, bring the arms behind the head, and move them from one side to the other.

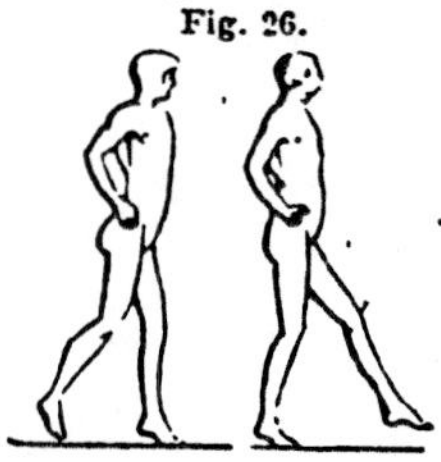

Fig. 25.

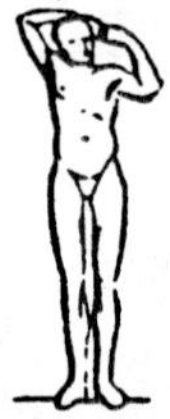

The action in fig. 26 is intended to act powerfully on the muscles of the leg and instep. Place the hands on the hips, the left leg in front, toe toward the ground; then jump forward on the right toe, both legs being kept quite straight.

Fig. 26.

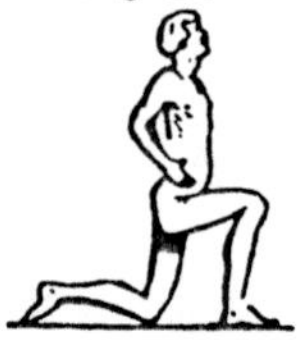

In fig. 27 the action exerts powerfully all the muscles of the leg and hip. Lift the left foot behind, bend the right knee, lower the body

Fig. 27.

Fig. 28.

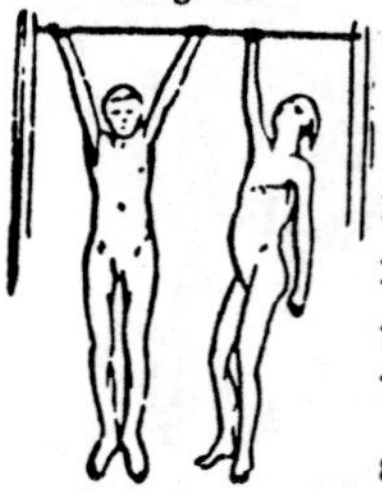

gradually, touch the ground with the left knee, and rise again.

In fig. 28 the action strongly exerts the muscles of the wrist and shoulder. Hang from the pole by one hand—first by the right, then by the left—several times alternately. Walking by the hands along the rounds of a ladder, where there is room, is an improvement on this exercise; and a semicircular ladder, on which the gymnast can ascend and descend, is better yet.

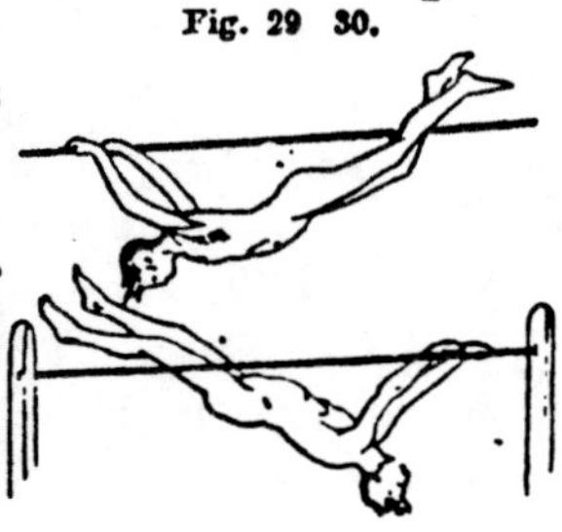

In figs. 29 and 30 the exercises are designed for putting the muscles of the arm and the chest to the utmost possible tension. In performing these evolutions the gymnast swings backward and forward a number of times, and finishes by jumping as he swings back, and comes down on the pole.

Fig. 29 30.

In fig. 31 the action calls the muscles of the wrists, arms, and shoulders into strong contraction. First throw the right leg over the pole; then, with a spring, bring up the right elbow; lastly, by another spring, bring up both arms straight, so as to sit across the pole.

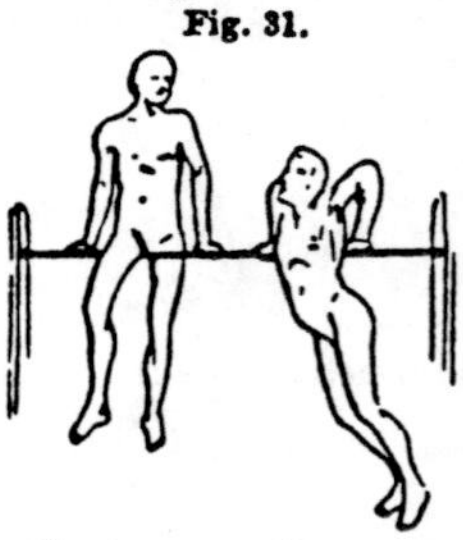

Fig. 31.

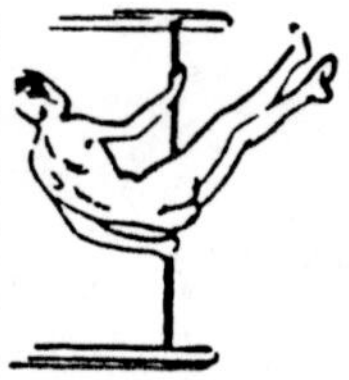

The action in fig. 32 throws nearly the whole effort upon the muscles of the wrist. Draw up the body as high as possible, and with a spring elevate both elbows at once, if possible, or one at a time; then rise gradually, the whole of the body being on one side of the pole; change the position of the hands, and come gradually over the pole till the feet touch the ground.

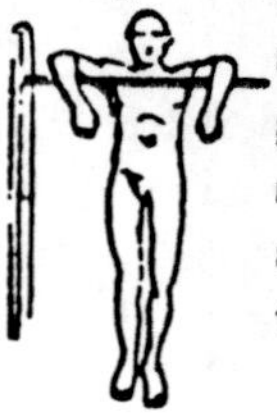

Fig. 32.

Fig. 33.

The action in fig. 33 brings the principal effort

on the muscles of the elbows and shoulders. Rise up as high as possible, and throw the arms over the pole, holding firmly by them.

The action in fig. 34 brings the principal effort on the elbow and shoulder of each arm alternately. Rise up as in the preceding case, and try to keep up the body by the right arm only, and then with the left.

Fig. 34.

For the special purpose of expanding the chest in cases of weak lungs or malformed chests, and in persons predisposed to consumption, the following exercises are excellent:

Fig. 35.

Fig. 35.—Bring the arms up quickly in front, as high as the shoulders—nails turned upward—then swing them forcibly backward, at the same time turning the nails backward, keeping the body perfectly upright.

After the above exercise is mastered, the next will call the respiratory muscles into still stronger play.

In the action in fig. 36 the elbows are to be drawn back so that the fists may be close to the sides; then throw the arms straight forward, and then back as before. When this action becomes easy and familiar, the succeeding ones are very easily acquired.

Fig. 36.

In the action in fig, 37 is a circular motion of the arms striking the wrists and palms to-

Fig. 37.

gether as the hands pass in front. It is one of the very best methods of enlarging the capacity of the air-cells of the lungs, by bringing the principal action upon the diaphragm and the pectoral muscles. These exercises may be improved upon by completely inflating the lungs with a full inspiration, and then holding the breath while half a dozen circular motions are made as rapidly as possible. And the best

13*

time to practice these gymnastics forcibly is just after the
morning bath, while the body is but partially dressed.   All
sedentary persons, and all the pent-up inhabitants of cities,
who do not enjoy the benefit of a walk before breakfast in
the open air, can find an excellent substitute in these muscular exercises.

Fig. 38.   Fig. 38 exercises the muscles of the lower extremities powerfully, and the abdominal muscles, with
the whole respiratory apparatus, moderately.   The
feet are to be brought close, the hands on the hips,
then rise on the toes; and jump on the   Fig. 39
toes, with the knees kept perfectly
straight.

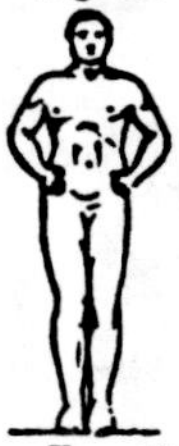

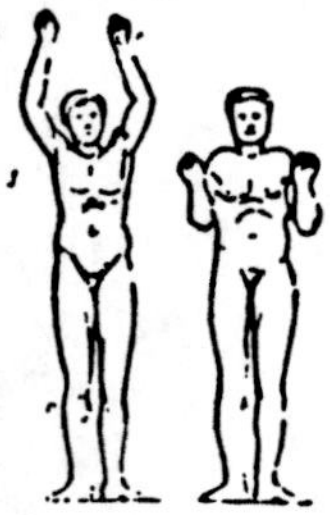

In the next action [fig. 39] the arms are
again brought into activity.   The fists are to
be brought up to the shoulders, the elbows
being close to the sides.   The arms are then to
be thrown upward, and then brought back
again to the previous position.   The action
may be extended to the abdominal muscles by, lastly, throwing the hands downward.

Fig. 40.   In fig. 40 the arms and muscles of the upper part of the
chest and back are more particularly called into action.
Raise the elbows to the height
of the shoulders,   Fig. 41.
with the fists on
the front of the
shoulders, the nails turned inward, and then
throw the arms forcibly back, the body being kept
perfectly upright.

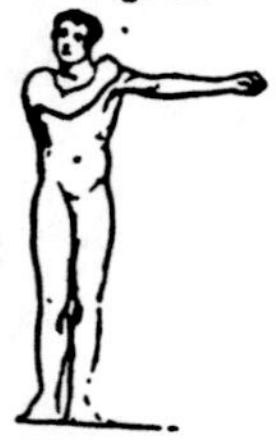

A still more powerful method of giving full
activity to all the muscles of the chest is represented in fig. 41.
Bring the right fist on the left shoulder; extend the left arm
in a line with the shoulder; throw the right arm toward the

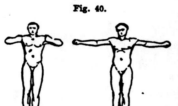

right side, nails toward the ground; then bring the left fist to the right.

Fig. 42.   The next action (fig. 42) calls into play those muscles of the back most intimately connected with respiration. Open the hands, then raise the arms sideways, and touch the back of the hands straight over the head.   Fig. 43.

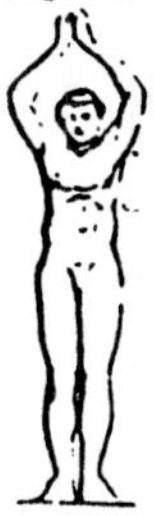

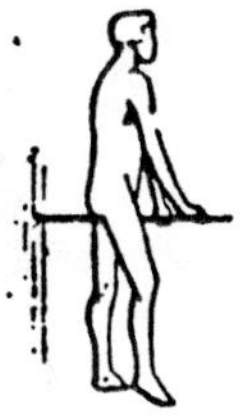

In figs. 43, 44, 45, and 46 are shown a variety of exercises calculated to act especially on the limbs, the upper extremities particularly. Some of them, as will be seen at a glance, act powerfully upon the muscles, ligaments, and fascia of the fingers, hands, and wrists, as in fig. 44; and motions testing the strength and action of the structure around the knee are seen in fig. 46.

Fig. 46.

Fig. 44.   Fig. 45.

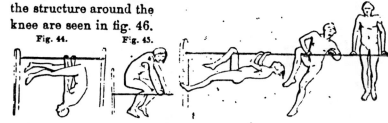

The flying steps, or giant strides [fig. 47,] are a very good and very amusing exercise for the arms and legs. A strong

Fig. 47.

post or mast is fixed firmly in the ground, on the top of which is an iron cap, revolving easily, to which the ropes are fastened. When in rapid motion, the pupils touch the ground hardly once to an entire revolution.

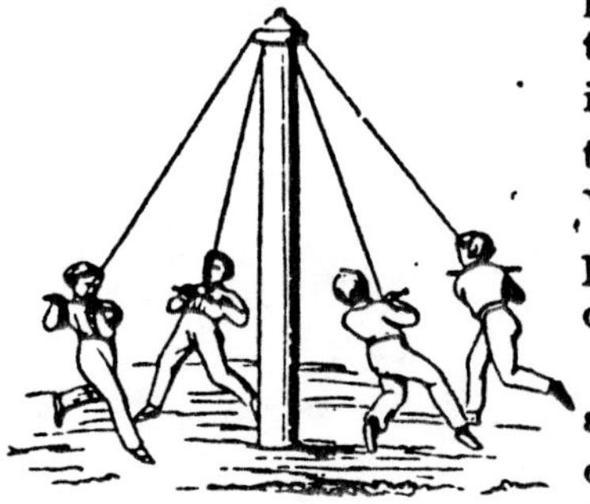

The parallel bars [fig. 48 and 49] are very conveniently constructed, and are calculated to act particularly on the joints

The Flying Steps.

of the wrist and shoulders, and generally on the whole respiratory system.

The body is first raised by the hands, and then swung alternately forward and backward; also pass along by moving the hands alternately, and then by moving both hands at once. The exercise may be varied in many ways, as throwing the limbs, and then the body, over the bars, lowering the body down until the elbows are level with the head, etc.

Fig. 48.   Fig. 49,

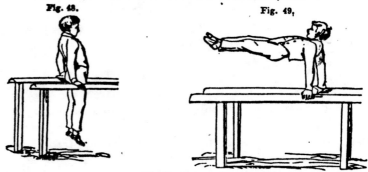

The Parallel Bars.

For young children of narrow, contracted chests, and weak digestive powers especially if they are attending school, this exercise is excellent.

FINIS.

nor show ~~nor sell a~~

I ~~For~~ $ hereby pledge that I will under no
circumstance give any ~~copied~~ text ~~the~~ which ^with^
Nina ~~provides me~~ gives to me to any other
person — not even to to ^provides^ ~~my family mem~~ any ~~one of~~
my family members nor ~~friends~~

I understand that this is the only condition under which
Nina is willing to provide me with

I am advised that ~~if I have any~~ unless

Signature: _____

I also understand that ~~Nina~~
any ^written^ information Nina may
give me is for educational
~~purposes only~~ — to inform me
and that Nina is in no way
recommending nor prescribing
any medical treatment. ~~to~~

I agree that in the event

Printed in the United States
863100001B

9 781564 598073